Urinary Dysfunction in Prostate Cancer

Jaspreet S. Sandhu

Editor

Urinary Dysfunction in Prostate Cancer

A Management Guide

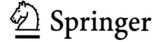

Editor
Jaspreet S. Sandhu
Department of Surgery
Urology Service
Memorial Sloan Kettering Cancer Center
New York, NY, USA

ISBN 978-3-319-23816-6   ISBN 978-3-319-23817-3   (eBook)
DOI 10.1007/978-3-319-23817-3

Library of Congress Control Number: 2015956175

Springer Cham Heidelberg New York Dordrecht London

Printed on acid-free paper

Springer International Publishing AG Switzerland is part of Springer Science+Business Media (www.springer.com)

Acknowledgements

I would like to acknowledge and thank the expert contributors who helped make this project a success. I know they sacrificed much family time in order to write their part of the manuscript and I appreciate their outstanding efforts. I would also like to thank my wife, Charan, and children, Amar and Rajan, for their love and understanding during this whole process.

Contents

Part I Introduction

1 **Introduction: Urinary Function Alterations in Men
with Prostate Cancer** 3
Gillian Stearns and Jaspreet S. Sandhu

Part II Adverse Events After Radical Prostatectomy

2 **Post-prostatectomy Incontinence Initial Evaluation** 15
Raveen Syan and Victor W. Nitti

3 **Urinary Incontinence: Conservative and Medical
Management and Injectable Therapy** 31
Hajar I. Ayoub and Ouida Lenaine Westney

4 **Urinary Dysfunction in Prostate Cancer: Male Slings** 53
Ricarda M. Bauer

5 **Artificial Urinary Sphincter: Patient Selection
and Surgical Technique** 71
Joseph J. Pariser, Andrew J. Cohen, Alexandre M. Rosen,
and Gregory T. Bales

6 **Troubleshooting and Optimizing Outcomes
After Artificial Urinary Sphincter** 93
Gillian Stearns and Jaspreet S. Sandhu

7 **Management of Vesicourethral Anastomotic Stricture** 101
Yuka Yamaguchi, Lee C. Zhao, and Allen T. Morey

8 **Rectourethral Fistula** 111
Jack M. Zuckerman and Kurt A. McCammon

9 **Reoperative Anti-incontinence Surgery** 125
Brian J. Linder and Daniel S. Elliott

Part III   Adverse Events After Radiotherapy

10   **Post-RT Urinary Incontinence and Stricture** 139
     Gillian Stearns and Laura Leddy

11   **A Case-Based Illustration of Urinary Symptoms**
     Following Radiation Therapy for Prostate Cancer 151
     Allison Polland, Michael S. Leapman, and Nelson N. Stone

Index 173

Contributors

Hajar I. Ayoub, M.D. Department of Urology, The University of Texas MD Anderson Cancer Center, Houston, TX, USA

Gregory T. Bales, M.D. Section of Urology, University of Chicago Medicine, Chicago, IL, USA

Ricarda M. Bauer, M.D. Department of Urology, Ludwig-Maximilians-University, Munich, Germany

Andrew J. Cohen, M.D. Section of Urology, University of Chicago Medicine, Chicago, IL, USA

Daniel S. Elliott, M.D. Department of Urology, Mayo Clinic, Rochester, MN, USA

Michael S. Leapman, M.D. Department of Urology, Mount Sinai Hospital, New York, NY, USA

Laura Leddy, M.D. Department of Surgery, Urology Service, Memorial Sloan Kettering Cancer Center, New York, NY, USA

Brian J. Linder, M.D. Department of Urology, Mayo Clinic, Rochester, MN, USA

Kurt A. McCammon, M.D., F.A.C.S. Department of Urology, Eastern Virginia Medical School, Norfolk, VA, USA

Allen T. Morey, M.D. Department of Urology, UT Southwestern Medical Center, Dallas, TX, USA

Victor W. Nitti, M.D. Department of Urology, Obstetrics and Gynecology, NYU Langone Medical Center, New York, NY, USA

Joseph J. Pariser, M.D. Section of Urology, University of Chicago Medicine, Chicago, IL, USA

Allison Polland, M.D. Department of Urology, Mount Sinai Hospital, New York, NY, USA

Alexandre M. Rosen, M.D. Specialists in Urology, Naples, FL, USA

Jaspreet S. Sandhu, M.D. Department of Surgery, Urology Service, Memorial Sloan Kettering Cancer Center, New York, NY, USA

Gillian Stearns, M.D. Department of Urology, University of Vermont, Burlington, VT, USA

Nelson N. Stone, M.D. Department of Urology, Mount Sinai Hospital, New York, NY, USA

Department of Urology and Radiation Oncology (RGS), Icahn School of Medicine at Mount Sinai, New York, NY, USA

Raveen Syan, M.D. Department of Urology, NYU Langone Medical Center, New York, NY, USA

Ouida Lenaine Westney, M.D. Department of Urology, The University of Texas MD Anderson Cancer Center, Houston, TX, USA

Yuka Yamaguchi, M.D. Department of Urology, NYU Langone Medical Center, New York, NY, USA

Lee C. Zhao, M.D., M.S. Department of Urology, New York University Langone Medical Center, New York, NY, USA

Jack M. Zuckerman, M.D. Department of Urology, Eastern Virginia Medical School, Norfolk, VA, USA

Part I

Introduction

Introduction: Urinary Function Alterations in Men with Prostate Cancer

Gillian Stearns and Jaspreet S. Sandhu

Introduction

The prostate gland plays an integral role in male reproduction during young adulthood. Its anatomic location, between the bladder and the membranous urethra, means that it is also an important part of the urinary voiding pathway and has a significant bystander effects on urinary function. The prevalence of urinary dysfunction, specifically lower urinary tract symptoms (LUTS) and urinary incontinence, increases as men age. LUTS in men is thought to be primarily a sequelae of benign prostatic hypertrophy (BPH), increases as men age as shown in multiple large longitudinal studies [1, 2]. As a rule of thumb, roughly half of men over the age of 50 suffer from some degree of LUTS. Urinary incontinence in community dwelling men, similarly, increases as men age. 11 % of men over the age of 65 without a history of prostate cancer or prostate surgery admit to suffering some degree of incontinence, increasing to 35 % in men over the age of 85 [3]. Prostate cancer

G. Stearns, M.D.
Department of Urology, University of Vermont, Burlington, VT, USA

J.S. Sandhu, M.D. (✉)
Department of Surgery, Urology Service, Memorial Sloan Kettering Cancer Center, 353 E 68St., New York, NY 10065, USA
e-mail: sandhuj@mskcc.org

afflicts elderly men and it is in this background that urinary function alterations after prostate cancer should be measured.

The control arm in one of the largest randomized trial performed to comparing radical prostatectomy as treatment for prostate cancer to an untreated "watchful waiting" cohort showed that untreated localized prostate cancer leads to slight worsening of urinary obstructive and irritative symptoms but not urinary incontinence [4].

It appears that LUTS due to prostate cancer in-situ behaves very much like LUTS due to BPH with the possibility of much faster progression. It is because of this reason that in men who have not had local treatment for prostate cancer, surgical modalities such as transurethral resection of the prostate (TURP) appear to be effective in relieving LUTS. Unfortunately, unlike TURP in the setting of BPH, TURP in the setting of locally advanced prostate cancer appears to be less durable likely due to continued tumor growth [5].

Urinary function alteration after local treatment for prostate cancer has been studied extensively, particularly in patients treated with radical prostatectomy or radiotherapy. Most studies show very similar results leading to an excellent understanding of the natural history of urinary function alterations after these treatments. Unfortunately, modalities such as cryotherapy, high-intensity focused ultrasound, focal therapy, and others do not have robust clinical data with respect to urinary adverse events.

Urinary Function After Radical Prostatectomy

Urinary function after radical prostatectomy changes dramatically in the short-term after radical prostatectomy [6]. Urinary incontinence, in particular, causes significant distress in men who have undergone radical prostatectomy [7].

Longitudinal studies show worsening urinary incontinence immediately after radical prostatectomy with subsequent improvement over the course of the next few months. Sanda et al. sought to qualify predictors of quality of life following patients who underwent treatment for prostate cancer and determine their effect on both the patient and partner. A total of 1201 patients were evaluated both pre- and post-treatment up to 24 months post treatment. Men who underwent prostatectomy reached a nadir in Quality of Life scores at 2 months post operatively which then improved over the following 24 months [6]. Irritative and obstructive scores improved to better than baseline over the study period. This finding was confirmed in another study by Pardo et al. A total of 435 patients were prospectively evaluated prior to treatment with prostatectomy, external beam radiotherapy or brachytherapy. Immediately post treatment, the prostatectomy cohort had worse incontinence quality of life scores at 36 months, but improved obstructive and irritative voiding symptoms. In patients with obstructive symptoms at baseline, 64 % of patients noted improvement above pretreatment [7]. Saranchuk et al. prospectively evaluated urinary function in 647 consecutive men undergoing radical prostatectomy and noted that full continence, defined as no pad use per day, was achieved in 87 % of men at 12 months which increased to 93 % at 2 years [8].

Multiple factors have been implicated in helping to achieve an earlier and more complete return to continence post-prostatectomy. Younger age has been shown to promote an earlier return to continence, as has preservation of the neurovascular bundles, lower body mass index (BMI), absence of anastomotic stricture, lower number of comorbidities, no prior radiotherapy for prostate cancer, and increasing membranous urethral length [9–11]. Grade, stage, and PSA were once thought to be associated with postoperative continence, but this may be attributed to nerve-sparing status instead [12]. Nerve-sparing status was found to decrease the median time to continence from 5.6 to 1.5 months in a study by Eastham et al. [10].

Multiple intraoperative maneuvers have also been described as well to help with postoperative continence. The role minimally invasive prostatectomy on subsequent incontinence remains unresolved.

Increasing age is an independent preoperative predictive factor for postoperative incontinence. Matsushita et al. evaluated 2849 patients and noted increasing age, higher ASA score, increasing BMI, and lower membranous urethral length were adverse independent predictors of subsequent continence recovery [11]. Age greater than 65 years of age has been associated with increased rates of incontinence and incomplete recovery of continence [9]. In a review of 581 consecutive patients, 91 % of patients were continent at 24 months and age less than 65 was the strongest correlate with recovery of continence [10]. In a prospective analysis by Licht et al., age greater than 65 years was an independent predictor of incontinence [13]. This reflects rates of continence in the aging male population as a whole. Anger et al. in a review of National Health and Nutrition Examination Survey have found that incontinence rates rose from an overall prevalence of 17 % in men younger than 60–31 % in men older than 85 [3].

Matsushita et al. showed an independent relationship between increasing BMI and subsequent incontinence, though there are some conflicting results [11]. Mulholland et al. demonstrated no association in body mass index and continence based on questionnaires related to voiding dysfunction over a 2 year period [14]. Conversely, Anast et al. showed that higher BMI was associated with worse urinary function, but not necessarily worsened quality of life after a review of the CaPSURE database [15]. This may have been associated with increased BMI leading to a higher rate of anastomotic stricture seen in a separate review of the CaPSURE data [16].

Smaller prostate volume has been suggested to result in improved continence rates; however, Eastham et al. found no association between prostate size and recovery of continence on multivariate analysis [10, 17]. Konety et al. reviewed the CaPSURE database for those patients with prostate volumes recorded and noted that prostate volumes less than 50 g were associated with improved continence rates; however, this difference normalized at 24 months postoperatively [17].

Newer modalities, such as laparoscopic or robotic prostatectomy, show similar results. Unfortunately, the difference in incontinence between open and MIS surgery has proven difficult to quantify because of the fact that very few surgeons offer both techniques contemporaneously. Furthermore, most comparisons have been between surgeons experienced in performing open surgery and those that have recently adopted MIS surgery, making conclusion problematic given effect of new technology and surgical learning curve.

Anastomotic Stricture After Radical Prostatectomy

Anastomotic stricture, or bladder neck contracture is a relatively uncommon, but well-known complication following radical prostatectomy. These patients tend to present in the first 6 months postoperatively [18, 19]. The economic impact of symptomatic urethral and anastomotic strictures is not insignificant, with one study documenting the cost at approximately $6000 per affected individual [20].

The rate of anastomotic stricture has been reported between 2.5 and 25.7 % in up to 62 % of patients who undergo radiotherapy [16, 18]. The wide range may be due in part to differences in data collection, patient population, surgeon practice patterns, and postoperative follow-up. These strictures are troublesome to manage, as they often require multiple procedures and intervention may lead to worsening of incontinence.

Risk factors for development of anastomotic stricture are similar to those seen for continued incontinence post prostatectomy and included age,

increased BMI, renal insufficiency, presence of postoperative leak or hematoma [18]. Individual surgeon technique and experience appear to greatly influence the development of strictures.

In a review of the SEER-Medicare linked database, Begg et al. noted a decreased rate of urinary complications, primarily anastomotic strictures, with higher volume surgeons [21]. Higher BMI and lower risk cancer were found to be associated with stricture formation upon review of the CaPSURE database [16].

With the rise in minimally invasive prostatectomy, a decrease in anastomotic strictures has been noted. Sandhu et al. found a roughly tenfold lower rate of anastomotic stricture in those patients undergoing MIS prostatectomy [18]. This was also noted in a SEER-Medicare linked database review by Hu et al. which showed that MIS prostatectomy was associated with 5.8 % rate of claims for bladder neck contracture versus 14 % for open [22]. In a retrospective review of 52 patients, Boroboroglu noted mucosal eversion during the vesicourethral anastomosis has been linked to decreased stricture formation and may present a possible explanation for the decreased stricture rate in minimally invasive prostatectomy. Other factors they noted on multivariate analysis included intraoperative blood loss, increased operative time, smoking, and coronary artery disease were also linked with development of bladder neck contracture [23].

The majority of these interventions are successful early; however, there is a subset of patients that require multiple interventions or further reconstruction. Most contractures are managed conservatively with dilation or transurethral incision, with success rates ranging between 50 and 87 % [19].

Urinary Function After Prostate Radiotherapy

Prostate radiotherapy is another option frequently used either alone or combined with androgen deprivation therapy (ADT) in patients with localized prostate cancer. Quality of life is often a factor in patient's decision making regarding which modality of treatment to undergo. A baseline voiding history should be undertaken as those patients with preexisting voiding dysfunction may experience worsening of their symptoms and should be counseled accordingly.

The Prostate Cancer Outcomes Study evaluated 3533 men and followed them for over 15 years to look at long-term functional outcomes of those patients undergoing treatment for localized prostate cancer. After 15 years, no difference was noted in the rates of urinary incontinence between those who underwent prostatectomy and those undergoing radiotherapy. Other voiding dysfunction was not assessed however [24]. Sanda noted an initial worsening of symptoms after external beam radiotherapy, albeit not as severe as seen post-surgery with an eventual return to baseline over 24 months. In those patients undergoing brachytherapy, symptoms did not return to baseline following treatment and patients were more likely to note persistent distress after 2 years. Eighteen percent of those patients undergoing brachytherapy reported moderate to severe distress at 12 months following initiation of treatment, compared to 11 % post radiotherapy and 7 % post prostatectomy [6]. A study by Ghadjar et al. also performed a prospective analysis of urinary toxicity following both external beam and brachytherapy. Most patients had a QoL score on the AUA Symptom Index of 2. This did not change throughout treatment as a whole. Twenty-eight percent of patients experienced acute Grade 2 toxicity, with 20 % continuing to have Grade 2–3 symptoms at more than 3 months beyond treatment. Grade 2 toxicity was described as urinary dysfunction requiring alpha blocker therapy. Grade 3 required catheterization or post-procedural transurethral resection of the prostate. Late Grade 3 toxicities were due primarily to urinary retention and were not associated in conjunction with Grade 2 toxicity [25]. At 3 years, the rate of urethral stenosis, incontinence, and hematuria were 6.6 %, 4.8 %, and 3.3 %, respectively, in a study by Fiorino [26].

Preoperative predictive factors include a PVR of greater than 100 cc, pre-procedural AUA symptom score of greater than 8, bladder outlet obstruction seen on urodynamics, prostate volume greater than 40 cc, and peak flow of less than 10 cc/s [27–29].

Large prostates were associated with persistent urinary toxicity in those patients undergoing both external beam and brachytherapy. In the study by Sanda et al., large prostate was defined as greater than 50 g [6].

At 1 year, 5 % of partners reported being bothered by the patient's incontinence. In the same cohort 7 % of partners were bothered by the patient's obstructive symptoms in those undergoing brachytherapy, compared to 3 % undergoing external beam radiotherapy [6].

Patients who present with urinary toxicity are managed medically initially, usually with alpha blocker therapy [30]. Anticholinergics have been used with some success for patients with persistent irritative voiding symptoms refractory to alpha blocker therapy alone [31]. Surgery may ultimately be indicated, but this may render the patient incontinent, necessitating careful and thorough counseling of the patient. Patient selection is also key in this situation. A history of a patient with new onset obstruction without prior voiding symptoms who is obstructed on urodynamic testing may benefit from resection. In a retrospective review of 38 patients who underwent TURP following brachytherapy, 18 % were incontinent post procedure. Median time to TURP was 11 months [32]. Incidence of rectourethral fistula is also higher and should be explained to patients as well. Aggressive anterior resection should be avoided to prevent development of pubovesical fistula [33].

Fistulae are late complications that result from instrumentation such as cystoscopy or colonoscopy in patients who have had prior radiation. Repair of rectourethral fistula is rendered more complicated secondary to the decreased vascularity of tissue surrounding the fistula and usually requires permanent diversion [34]. This is similar to data seen for pubovesical fistulae. Patients typically presented with urethral stricture and underwent endoscopic treatment. Conservative management was typically unsuccessful with most patients undergoing eventual cystectomy [33].

Radiation may also be used as a salvage therapy in patients who have undergone first line treatments for their prostate cancer. In a recent meta-analysis grade 3–4 toxicity was found to be significantly higher in the salvage brachytherapy group, occurring in 12.9 % of patients. Incontinence was reported in 6.2 and 3.1 % developed recto-urinary fistula [35]. Tharp et al. however reported toxicity of urethral necrosis and incontinence in 29 % of their cohort with a median of 58 month follow-up [36].

Emerging Topics in Urinary Dysfunction After Prostate Cancer

Urinary Function Recovery After Prostate Cancer Ablation

New data is emerging as short term studies arise regarding voiding dysfunction following whole gland ablation. The COLD database is a database of all men undergoing cryotherapy, both focal and whole gland, in both primary and salvage settings. 4099 patients underwent whole gland cryoablation between 1999 and 2007. In the report of complications 65/2099 (3.1 %) reported de novo incontinence. 18/2099 (0.4 %) developed rectourethral fistula, and 34/2177 (1.6 %) had urinary retention persisting more than 30 days post procedure [37]. A recent study evaluating urodynamic outcomes saw decreased bladder compliance and de novo overactive bladder in 10 % of patients at 3 months post-procedure, improving by 6 months follow-up. At 6 months, the cohort showed decreased Pdet, and Qmax on uroflowmetry. Those patients with large prostates continued to have voiding dysfunction at the 6 month procedure period [38]. Another study with a median of 27 months follow-up showed urethral stricture formation requiring dilation in 13.8 % of patients. Bladder neck incision was required in 9.2 %. Before treatment 73.3 % of patients did not leak, post treatment 55 % of patients did not leak. 2.7 % of patients did not require pads pretreatment, increasing to 9 % following treatment [39].

Whole gland cryoablation has also been used as both a primary and salvage treatment for prostate cancer. In the early postoperative phase, voiding dysfunction worsened, yet returned to baseline by 12 months post procedure. These symptoms were noted to be better than the brachytherapy cohort [40]. Kvorning Ternov et al. found that in 30 patients undergoing salvage cryotherapy 11 (36.6 %) had Grade 1–2 urinary incontinence, another 3 (10 %) had grade 3–4. Three (10 %) ultimately developed a urethral stricture and one (3 %) developed a fistula 4.5 years post procedure [41]. The COLD database showed a higher rate of urinary complications as compared to those undergoing whole gland cryotherapy for primary treatment of their prostate cancer when cryotherapy was performed in a salvage setting. Incontinence rates were 12.3 % (33/299), rectourethral fistula occurred in 1.5 % (5/194), and persistent urinary retention occurred in 12/282 (4.3 %) [37].

High-intensity focused ultrasound (HIFU) is also being used as both whole gland and focal therapy for localized prostate cancer. Crouzet et al. evaluated the oncologic outcomes and morbidity of 1002 patients who underwent HIFU for treatment of their prostate cancer between 1997 and 2009. Rates of urinary complications decreased with change from the prototype model to newer versions of the ultrasound machine. Prior to 2000, 15/63 (23.8 %) of patients had grade 1 stress urinary incontinence, compared to 42/287 (14.6 %) between 2005 and 2009. 4/63 had Grade 2–3 incontinence prior to 2000 while only 9/287 (3.1 %) had grade 2–3 incontinence. Acute urinary retention was seen in 10.2 % of 1002 patients and bladder outlet obstruction was seen in 16.6 % (166/1002). Late complications included fistula and urethral stenosis, occurring in 90/1002 patients (9 %) and 4/1002(0.4 %), respectively [42]. Rectourethral fistula formation was seen in only patients who had undergone salvage HIFU and had significant comorbidities or prior radiation history.

Urinary retention is thought initially to be due to edema following the procedure. Prolonged obstruction may be secondary to sloughing of necrotic debris. Due to this high rate of urinary retention following HIFU, transurethral resection of the prostate (TURP) is frequently used in patients with larger prostates to help prevent obstructive symptoms postoperatively [43].

In the study by Crouzet et al., after 2000, all patients with a prostate volume of greater than 30 g underwent TURP immediately prior to their HIFU treatment. Chaussy et al. compared to patients who underwent HIFU alone with those who underwent TURP immediately prior to HIFU. 96 patients underwent HIFU alone compared to 175 who underwent HIFU and TURP. At 3 months post-HIFU, Quality of Life subscore on IPSS increased from 1.3 to 2.36 for HIFU alone versus 2.06 to 1.85 with HIFU and TURP. Suprapubic catheter remained for a median of 40 days, as compared to 13.7 days in those patients undergoing TURP and HIFU. Urinary tract infections were noted in 47.9 % in those undergoing HIFU alone, compared to 11.4 in those with both procedures. 27.1 % of patients required further deobstruction procedures, either removal of necrotic debris or dilation for bladder neck contracture, compared to 8 % of the TURP and HIFU [42].

Voiding Dysfunction in Men Following Focal Therapy

Given the morbidity following whole gland prostate cancer treatment, interest persists regarding the possibility of focal therapy for localized prostate cancer. The focus of focal therapy is to eradicate the index tumor while preserving nearby structures, such as bladder and rectum, decreasing rates of urinary, bowel and sexual dysfunction post procedure. Long term data is lacking for most of these treatment modalities. Review of the COLD registry evaluating focal cryotherapy found limited urinary morbidity, reporting rectourethral fistula in 1/1160 patients. Urinary continence was maintained in 499 of 507 (98.4 %) with urinary retention persisting 1 month from therapy reported in 1.1 % (6/518) [37]. Focal HIFU was initially used as salvage treatment for patients who had failed primary treatment, usually with radiation as the primary treatment modality. The first study looking at outcomes of focal HIFU looked at 39 patients who underwent salvage therapy between 2004 and 2009. At a median follow-up of 17 months, 64 % reported being pad and leak free with 87.2 % being pad free. One rectoure-

thral fistula occurred [44]. A further study looked at 20 patients undergoing hemigland HIFU at up to 1 year follow-up. 18/20 (90 %) were leak-free and pad free. At baseline, nine reported mild urinary symptoms and ten reported moderate urinary symptoms. By the end of 12 months, 16 reported mild urinary symptoms with 4 reporting moderate and no severe urinary issues. Quality of life remained unchanged throughout the follow-up period [45].

Voiding Dysfunction in Men with Locally Advanced Prostate Cancer

Those patients who present with locally advanced prostate cancer may experience voiding dysfunction, usually in the form of obstruction. Little data exists as to the role of pharmacotherapy in this cohort. Those patients who undergo initiation of hormone deprivation may experience relief of their symptoms. In a study 35 patients with locally invasive prostate cancer who presented with urinary retention were randomized to either orchiectomy or transurethral resection of the prostate for treatment of their obstructive symptoms. Retention resolved in 24/35 patients (68.6 %) with orchiectomy alone [46]. Historically, TURP was not performed for relief of obstruction due to concern for acceleration of the disease process. In a review of 184 patients, Levine et al. sought to determine the impact of TURP on disease progression and cancer specific mortality. In locally advanced cancer (Whitmore-Jewett stage C/D), there was no difference in disease progression between the TURP group and the control. For those patients with organ confined disease (Whitmore-Jewett stage B), disease specific mortality was significantly higher in the group undergoing TURP [47]. A review of the SEER database showed 2742/29361 patients underwent TURP following their prostate cancer diagnosis. The outcome of interest was markers of disease progression, defined as orchiectomy or procedures indicating worsening urinary obstruction. Those patients that underwent TURP were more likely to undergo orchiectomy; however, the authors felt this was likely due to the severity of disease rather than the surgery itself [48]. TURP does appear to be effective in relieving urinary symptoms due to obstruction from prostate cancer. In a retrospective review of 24 palliative TURPs, Crain et al. found an improvement in IPSS from 21.1 to 11 when patients underwent resection. They were more likely to fail voiding trial than the cohort of patients undergoing resection for benign disease and more likely to require reoperation for repeat obstruction [49].

Conclusion

Treatment of prostate cancer is associated with changes in voiding function. While much is known about the effects of radical prostatectomy and radiation therapy on urinary function, treatment for prostate cancer continues to evolve. As such, research regarding the natural history of urinary function after these newer treatment modalities continues and patient counseling changes accordingly.

References

1. Garraway WM, Collins GN, Lee RJ. High prevalence of benign prostatic hypertrophy in the community. Lancet. 1991;338(8765):469–71.
2. Arrighi HM, Metter EJ, Guess HA, Fozzard JL. Natural history of benign prostatic hyperplasia and risk of prostatectomy. The Baltimore Longitudinal Study of Aging. Urology. 1991;38(1 Suppl):4–8.
3. Anger JT, Saigal CS, Stothers L, Thom DH, Rodríguez LV, Litwin MS, Urologic Diseases of America Project. The prevalence of urinary incontinence among community dwelling men: results from the National Health and Nutrition Examination survey. J Urol. 2006;176(5):2103–8.
4. Johansson E, Steineck G, Holmberg L, Johansson JE, Nyberg T, Ruutu M, Bill-Axelson A, SPCG-4 Investigators. Long-term quality-of-life outcomes after radical prostatectomy or watchful waiting: the Scandinavian Prostate Cancer Group-4 randomised trial. Lancet Oncol. 2011;12(9):891–9.
5. Anast JW, Andriole GL, Grubb II RL. Managing the local complications of locally advanced prostate cancer. Curr Urol Rep. 2007;8(3):211–6.
6. Sanda MG, Dunn RL, Michalski J, Sandler HM, Northouse L, Hembroff L, Lin X, Greenfield TK,

7. Litwin MS, Saigal CS, Mahadevan A, Klein E, Kibel A, Pisters LL, Kuban D, Kaplan I, Wood D, Ciezki J, Shah N, Wei JT. Quality of life and satisfaction with outcome among prostate-cancer survivors. N Engl J Med. 2008;358(12):1250–61.
7. Pardo Y, Guedea F, Aguiló F, Fernández P, Macías V, Mariño A, Hervás A, Herruzo I, Ortiz MJ, Ponce de León J, Craven-Bratle J, Suárez JF, Boladeras A, Pont À, Ayala A, Sancho G, Martínez E, Alonso J, Ferrer M. Quality-of-life impact of primary treatments for localized prostate cancer in patients without hormonal treatment. J Clin Oncol. 2010;28(31):4687–96.
8. Saranchuk JW, Kattan MW, Elkin E, Touijer AK, Scardino PT, Eastham JA. Achieving optimal outcomes after radical prostatectomy. J Clin Oncol. 2005;23(18):4146–51.
9. Sandhu JS, Eastham JA. Factors predicting early return of continence after radical prostatectomy. Curr Urol Rep. 2010;11(3):191–7.
10. Eastham JA, Kattan MW, Rogers E, Goad JR, Ohori M, Boone TB, Scardino PT. Risk factors for urinary incontinence after radical prostatectomy. J Urol. 1996;156(5):1707–13.
11. Matsushita K, Kent MT, Vickers AJ, von Bodman C, Bernstein M, Touijer KA, Coleman JA, Laudone VT, Scardino PT, Eastham JA, Akin O, Sandhu JS. Preoperative predictive model of recovery of urinary continence after radical prostatectomy. BJU Int. 2015. doi:10.1111/bju.13087.
12. Burkhard FC, Kessler TM, Fleischmann A, Thalmann GN, Schumacher M, Studer UE. Nerve sparing open radical retropubic prostatectomy--does it have an impact on urinary continence? J Urol. 2006;176(1):189–95.
13. Licht MR, Klein EA, Tuason L, Levin H. Impact of bladder neck preservation during radical prostatectomy on continence and cancer control. Urology. 1994;44(6):883–7.
14. Mulholland TL, Huynh PN, Huang RR, Wong C, Diokno AC, Peters KM. Urinary incontinence after radical retropubic prostatectomy is not related to patient body mass index. Prostate Cancer Prostatic Dis. 2006;9(2):153–9.
15. Anast JW, Sadetsky N, Pasta DJ, Bassett WW, Latini D, DuChane J, Chan JM, Cooperberg MR, Carroll PR, Kane CJ. The impact of obesity on health related quality of life before and after radical prostatectomy (data from CaPSURE). J Urol. 2005;173(4):1132–8.
16. Elliott SP, Meng MV, Elkin EP, McAninch JW, Duchane J, Carroll PR, CaPSURE Investigators. Incidence of urethral stricture after primary treatment for prostate cancer: data From CaPSURE. J Urol. 2007;178(2):529–34.
17. Konety BR, Sadetsky N, Carroll PR, CaPSURE Investigators. Recovery of urinary continence following radical prostatectomy: the impact of prostate volume--analysis of data from the CaPSURE Database. J Urol. 2007;177(4):1423–5.
18. Sandhu JS, Gotto GT, Herran LA, Scardino PT, Eastham JA, Rabbani F. Age, obesity, medical comorbidities and

surgical technique are predictive of symptomatic anastomotic strictures after contemporary radical prostatectomy. J Urol. 2011;185(6):2148–52.

19. Ramirez D, Simhan J, Hudak SJ, Morey AF. Standardized approach for the treatment of refractory bladder neck contractures. Urol Clin North Am. 2013;40(3):371–80.

20. Santucci RA, Joyce GF, Wise M. Male urethral stricture disease. J Urol. 2007;177(5):1667–74.

21. Begg CB, Riedel ER, Bach PB, Kattan MW, Schrag D, Warren JL, Scardino PT. Variations in morbidity after radical prostatectomy. N Engl J Med. 2002;346(15):1138–44.

22. Hu JC, Gu X, Lipsitz SR, Barry MJ, D'Amico AV, Weinberg AC, Keating NL. Comparative effectiveness of minimally invasive vs open radical prostatectomy. JAMA. 2009;302(14):1557–64.

23. Borboroglu PG, Sands JP, Roberts JL, Amling CL. Risk factors for vesicourethral anastomotic stricture after radical prostatectomy. Urology. 2000;56(1): 96–100.

24. Resnick MJ, Koyama T, Fan KH, Albertsen PC, Goodman M, Hamilton AS, Hoffman RM, Potosky AL, Stanford JL, Stroup AM, Van Horn RL, Penson DF. Long-term functional outcomes after treatment for localized prostate cancer. N Engl J Med. 2013; 368(5):436–45.

25. Ghadjar P, Jackson A, Spratt DE, Oh JH, Munck af Rosenschöld P, Kollmeier M, Yorke E, Hunt M, Deasy JO, Zelefsky MJ. Patterns and predictors of amelioration of genitourinary toxicity after high-dose intensity-modulated radiation therapy for localized prostate cancer: implications for defining postradiotherapy urinary toxicity. Eur Urol. 2013; 64(6):931–8.

26. Fiorino C, Cozzarini C, Rancati T, Briganti A, Cattaneo GM, Mangili P, Di Muzio NG, Calandrino R. Modelling the impact of fractionation on late urinary toxicity after postprostatectomy radiation therapy. Int J Radiat Oncol Biol Phys. 2014;90(5):1250–7.

27. Gelblum DY, Potters L, Ashley R, Waldbaum R, Wang XH, Leibel S. Urinary morbidity following ultrasound-guided transperineal prostate seed implantation. Int J Radiat Oncol Biol Phys. 1999;45(1): 59–67.

28. Beekman M, Merrick GS, Butler WM, Wallner KE, Allen ZA, Galbreath RW. Selecting patients with pretreatment postvoid residual urine volume less than 100 mL may favorably influence brachytherapy-related urinary morbidity. Urology. 2005;66(6): 1266–70.

29. Martens C, Pond G, Webster D, McLean M, Gillan C, Crook J. Relationship of the International Prostate Symptom score with urinary flow studies, and catheterization rates following 125I prostate brachytherapy. Brachytherapy. 2006;5(1):9–13.

30. Elshaikh MA, Ulchaker JC, Reddy CA, Angermeier KW, Klein EA, Chehade N, Altman A, Ciezki JP. Prophylactic tamsulosin (Flomax) in patients undergoing prostate 125I brachytherapy for prostate carcinoma: final report of a double-blind placebo-controlled randomized study. Int J Radiat Oncol Biol Phys. 2005;62(1):164–9.

31. Bittner N, Merrick GS, Brammer S, Niehaus A, Wallner KE, Butler WM, Allen ZA, Galbreath RW. Role of trospium chloride in brachytherapy-related detrusor overactivity. Urology. 2008;71(3):460–4.

32. Kollmeier MA, Stock RG, Cesaretti J, Stone NN. Urinary morbidity and incontinence following transurethral resection of the prostate after brachytherapy. J Urol. 2005;173(3):808–12.

33. Matsushita K, Ginsburg L, Mian BM, De E, Chughtai BI, Bernstein M, Scardino PT, Eastham JA, Bochner BH, Sandhu JS. Pubovesical fistula: a rare complication after treatment of prostate cancer. Urology. 2012;80(2):446–51.

34. Linder BJ, Umbreit EC, Larson D, Dozois EJ, Thapa P, Elliott DS. Effect of prior radiotherapy and ablative therapy on surgical outcomes for the treatment of rectourethral fistulas. J Urol. 2013;190(4):1287–91.

35. Parekh A, Graham PL, Nguyen PL. Cancer control and complications of salvage local therapy after failure of radiotherapy for prostate cancer: a systematic review. Semin Radiat Oncol. 2013;23(3):222–34.

36. Tharp M, Hardacre M, Bennett R, Jones WT, Stuhldreher D, Vaught J. Prostate high-dose-rate brachytherapy as salvage treatment of local failure after previous external or permanent seed irradiation for prostate cancer. Brachytherapy. 2008;7(3):231–6.

37. Ward JF, Jones JS. Focal cryotherapy for localized prostate cancer: a report from the national Cryo On-Line Database (COLD) Registry. BJU Int. 2012;109(11):1648–54.

38. Mearini L, D'Urso L, Collura D, Nunzi E, Muto G, Porena M. High-intensity focused ultrasound for the treatment of prostate cancer: a prospective trial with long-term follow-up. Scand J Urol. 2014;8:1–8.

39. Berge V, Dickinson L, McCartan N, Hindley RG, Diep LM, Emberton M, Ahmed HU. Morbidity associated with primary high intensity focused ultrasound and redo high intensity focused ultrasound for localized prostate cancer. J Urol. 2014;191(6):1764–9.

40. Hubosky SG, Fabrizio MD, Schellhammer PF, Barone BB, Tepera CM, Given RW. Single center experience with third-generation cryosurgery for management of organ-confined prostate cancer: critical evaluation of short-term outcomes, complications, and patient quality of life. J Endourol. 2007;21(12):1521–31.

41. Kvorning Ternov K, Krag Jakobsen A, Bratt O, Ahlgren G. Salvage cryotherapy for local recurrence after radiotherapy for prostate cancer. Scand J Urol. 2015;49(2):115–9.

42. Crouzet S, Chapelon JY, Rouvière O, Mege-Lechevallier F, Colombel M, Tonoli-Catez H, Martin X, Gelet A. Whole-gland ablation of localized prostate cancer with high-intensity focused ultrasound: oncologic outcomes and morbidity in 1002 patients. Eur Urol. 2014;65(5):907–14.

43. Chaussy C, Thüroff S. The status of high-intensity focused ultrasound in the treatment of localized prostate cancer and the impact of a combined resection. Curr Urol Rep. 2003;4(3):248–52.

44. Ahmed HU, Cathcart P, McCartan N, Kirkham A, Allen C, Freeman A, Emberton M. Focal salvage therapy for localized prostate cancer recurrence after external beam radiotherapy: a pilot study. Cancer. 2012;118(17):4148–55.

45. Ahmed HU, Freeman A, Kirkham A, Sahu M, Scott R, Allen C, Van der Meulen J, Emberton M. Focal therapy for localized prostate cancer: a phase I/II trial. J Urol. 2011;185(4):1246–54.

46. Fleischmann JD, Catalona WJ. Endocrine therapy for bladder outlet obstruction from carcinoma of the prostate. J Urol. 1985;134(3):498–500.

47. Levine ES, Cisek VJ, Mulvihill MN, Cohen EL. Role of transurethral resection in dissemination of cancer of prostate. Urology. 1986;28(3):179–83.

48. Krupski TL, Stukenborg GJ, Moon K, Theodorescu D. The relationship of palliative transurethral resection of the prostate with disease progression in patients with prostate cancer. BJU Int. 2010;106(10): 1477–83.

49. Crain DS, Amling CL, Kane CJ. Palliative transurethral prostate resection for bladder outlet obstruction in patients with locally advanced prostate cancer. J Urol. 2004;171(2 Pt 1):668–71.

Part II

Adverse Events After Radical Prostatectomy

Raveen Syan and Victor W. Nitti

Post-prostatectomy Incontinence: Introduction

Incidence

Urinary incontinence is a relatively common complication following radical prostatectomy (RP) with a wide range of reportedincidence, from 2 to 87 % [1]. Some of this variability may be attributable to differences between clinicians in defining and classifying post-prostatectomy incontinence (PPI) [2]. A group that examined patient-reported outcomes found 33 % of men had urinary incontinence requiring the use of protective devices such as pads, diapers, rubber pants and clamps [3]. Severe incontinence, as defined by either total incontinence or frequent urinary leakage, has been reported to be as high as 8.4 % [2].

It has been well recognized that there is a time-dependent relationship to return of continence after prostatectomy. Incontinence rates decline over time, and generally patients establish their continence baseline status 1–2 years following surgery [4]. Early incontinence is common, while return to continence at 1 year has been reported to be greater than 90 % [5, 6]. Thus it is generally recommended that patients not undergo an invasive anti-incontinence therapy until 6–12 months after surgery to allow for a baseline status to be achieved prior to intervention. Some groups recommend a trial of conservative therapy including pelvic floor physiotherapy first [4]. However, many groups have shown that the majority of patients will have reached baseline continence by 6 months [7]. Penson et al. followed 1213 patients who underwent RP and found that rates of severe urinary incontinence (frequent urinary leakage or no control) peaked at 6 months and steadily declined at 2 years following surgery to 10 % [8]. Goluboff et al. determined that 92 % of their patients reached their final continence status at 6 months [9] and Smither et al. demonstrated that the majority of patients who achieved continence did so as early as 18 weeks postoperatively, with little significant change in functional status until 54 weeks [10].

Another caveat to early observation is that patients with severe early urinary incontinence are more likely to have long-term incontinence. Vickers et al. examined patients who underwent a radical prostatectomy and evaluated the number of pads required at 3, 6, 9, and 12 months, and then reevaluated urinary continence status at 2 years. They found that patients requiring one or two pads at 6 months had a low probability of

R. Syan, M.D.
Department of Urology, NYU Langone Medical Center, New York, NY, USA

V.W. Nitti, M.D. (✉)
Department of Urology, Obstetrics and Gynecology, NYU Langone Medical Center, 150 East 32nd Street, 2nd Floor, New York, NY 10016, USA
e-mail: victor.nitti@nyumc.org

© Springer International Publishing Switzerland 2016
J.S. Sandhu (ed.), *Urinary Dysfunction in Prostate Cancer*, DOI 10.1007/978-3-319-23817-3_2

being pad free at 2 years (50 and 36 %, respectively) [11]. This group suggests that severe urinary incontinence even within the first year of surgery is a predictor for poor long-term function, and should be considered for earlier identification and possible intervention.

The benefit of early intervention has been studied. Schneider et al. compared PPI patients with SUI who underwent early periurethral bulking procedure at a mean time of 23 days postoperatively with patients treated at 26 months postoperatively. They found that short-term continence results were higher in the early intervention group, however long-term results were similar [12]. Jones et al. found similar results when comparing intervention with the urethral sling, in that early intervention provided improved short-term but equivalent long-term results [13].

Based on the available clinical data and or own experience, we generally wait about 12 months prior to evaluation and surgical treatment for patients with mild to moderate incontinence, especially if they are noting continued improvement. If a patient is still improving at 12 months, it may be prudent to delay surgical therapy a bit longer. For patients with severe incontinence that is not improving, evaluation and surgical intervention is considered at 6 months. This is dependent of course on the degree of bother to the patient and his willingness to undergo a surgical procedure.

Pathophysiology

The internal urethral sphincter (IUS) lies at the bladder base and is composed of smooth muscle, while the external urethral sphincter (EUS) is composed of skeletal muscle and is under volitional control. The IUS has both longitudinal and circular muscular layers, where continence is mediated by noradrenaline from sympathetic fibers acting on $\alpha 1$-adrenoceptors to cause contraction of the circular smooth muscle and relaxation of the longitudinal smooth muscle via B3-adrenergic receptors. During voiding, the longitudinal smooth muscle contracts while the circular smooth muscle relaxes via nitric oxide and acetylcholine release from parasympathetic

fibers, allowing for bladder emptying. The EUS is composed of striated muscle, where contraction and relaxation is mediated via the pudendal nerve [4].

The urinary sphincteric mechanism can also be divided into proximal and distal sphincter. The proximal urinary sphincter is formed by the bladder neck, prostate, and prostatic urethra to the verumontanum, under both parasympathetic and sympathetic control. During a radical prostatectomy, the proximal urinary sphincter is effectively removed. Continence is therefore dependent upon the distal urethral sphincter. This is comprised of the distal EUS, the prostatomembranous urethra, and the supporting musculature and fascia of the pelvis [14]. Therefore, incontinence following radical prostatectomy is most often attributable to dysfunction of the distal urethral sphincter. This can occur as a result of direct injury to the DUS, damage to its nerve supply or supporting structures, or preexisting dysfunction. Intraoperative preservation of this tissue is important to preserve continence [15].

The etiology of post-prostatectomy incontinence (PPI) is most often attributable to sphincteric incompetence (SI) that exists with or without bladder dysfunction in about 95 % of cases [1, 16–19]. Isolated bladder dysfunction, such as detrusor overactivity or decreased bladder compliance is a rare cause of post-prostatectomy incontinence. Groutz et al. performed urodynamic evaluation of 83 men with PPI and found 33 % had bladder dysfunction; however, only 7 % had bladder dysfunction as an isolated cause for PPI [16]. Some groups have reported rates of bladder dysfunction as a sole cause for PPI as low as 3 % [20], while concomitant sphincter and bladder dysfunction accounts for 34–45 % of patients with PPI [4]. De novo bladder dysfunction may be due to intraoperative bladder denervation or outlet obstruction. Giannantoni et al. found that de novo decreased bladder compliance and detrusor underactivity shown on urodynamics 1 month after radical prostatectomy had improved and resolved at 8 months in the majority of patients [21]. Sphincteric incompetence overall remains the primary cause of PPI, believed due to direct damage and manipulation intraoperatively [4].

When patients have combined urinary incontinence and a decreased force of stream, scarring leading to urethral stricture disease should be the suspected cause [22].

Following a radical prostatectomy, urinary continence is dependent upon on the distal urethral sphincter. Sphincteric incompetence accounts for approximately 95 % of post-prostatectomy incontinence, though concurrent bladder dysfunction may be present in 30 % of cases. Isolated bladder dysfunction is a rare cause of PPI. Urethral or anastomotic stricture should be suspected in patients with obstruction voiding patterns or a decreased force of stream.

Factors That Drive Treatment

With the wide range in degree and type of incontinence that occurs following a radical prostatectomy, several factors may influence a patient's desire to undergo either conservative or invasive treatment. For some patients, PPI can have a significant effect on quality of life (QoL). Fowler et al. published results from a Medicare survey and found that leakage of urine requiring use of protective pads had a more significant effect on patient's quality of life than sexual dysfunction, and patients were significantly less likely to report satisfaction with surgical treatment [23]. Greater degree of incontinence not only worsens patient reported QoL; it also influences the degree of bother they experience, which then influences their desire for further intervention [4]. Overall, studies suggest that while mild incontinence can be acceptable to patients in exchange for cancer control, requiring regular use of protective devices or pads has a significant influence on patient QoL and may influence desire for further treatment [7, 23].

The type of incontinence also influences patient decision to undergo intervention. Stress urinary incontinence is most common in the early postoperative period and has been well demonstrated to improve over time. This may guide clinicians to counsel patients to continue conservative measures prior to pursuing more invasive options [4].

Patient's desire for cure can also influence counseling and treatment options. There are no curative medical interventions, though medications such asduloxetine have been shown to improve mild to moderate incontinence [24]. A cure for PPI can be achieved with more invasive measures such as surgical interventions; however, these interventions have their own risks and potential effects on symptoms and quality of life.

All of the above factors are important in determining evaluation and intervention for PPI. But in reality it is always an individual patient's decision based on the personal degree of bother. While the degree of incontinence will influence the type of treatment recommended, it is the degree of bother that drives the decision to intervene at all. There are general trends, but the bottom line is that some men are highly bothered by relatively mild incontinence, while others who have severe incontinence may not be "bothered" at all. It is also important that patients have reasonable expectations from treatments, especially those who are highly bothered by mild incontinence.

Patient Risk Factors for PPI

There are a number of recognized preoperative risk factors that increase the rate of PPI. By identifying those patients at increased risk for PPI, preoperative counseling and postoperative management can be better tailored to the individual patient.

Wallerstedt et al. evaluated 1529 patients who underwent a radical prostatectomy for clinically localized prostate cancer with questionnaires 3 months prior to surgery and 12 months after surgery. Incontinence was defined as requiring more than one pad daily to control urination. This group found that age and presence of preoperative urinary leakage were significant predictors of PPI. Prior transurethral resection of prostate for obstructive symptoms was not significantly associated with PPI [25]. Kim et al. also found that age was a significant predictor of PPI, where younger patients tended to have higher rates of early continence recovery [26], and Novara et al.

found that younger age was an independent predictor of continence at 12 months [27]. Catalona's group examined influence of age on return of continence in 1325 men 18 months postoperatively and found that men younger than 70 had continence rates of 92–97 %, while men in their 70s had a significantly lower continence rate of 87 % [28].

Evidence of sphincteric incompetence preoperatively has been demonstrated to increase the risk of postoperative urinary incontinence, primarily resulting in stress urinary incontinence (SUI). Preoperative bladder dysfunction such as detrusor overactivity or an acontractile bladder has also been shown to be a risk factor for PPI [15].

Song et al. performed pelvic MRI imaging on 94 patients prior to undergoing a radical prostatectomy and evaluated the association between the integrity of the pelvic floor muscles, measured by thickness of the pelvic diaphragm as well as ratio of levator ani thickness to prostate volume, and urinary continence. They defined incontinence as any unwanted leakage of urine and found that these measures of pelvic floor integrity were associated with earlier recovery of continence after surgery [29]. Prostate size has not been clearly shown in the literature to influence continence status after prostatectomy, and this group suggests that the presence of pelvic support is more significant than the absolute size of the prostate.

A number of groups have evaluated the influence of obesity on PPI. Xu et al. performed a meta-analysis of 13 observational studies and found that obese patients were significantly more likely to have PPI [30]. They hypothesize that this may be due to intraoperative factors, such as excessive peri-prostatic fat limiting visualization and manipulation of urethra and neurovascular bundle, as well as postoperative factors such as increased pressure on the bladder and pelvic floor.

Stage of disease has not been conclusively related to rates of PPI, though a more advanced stage of disease may affect the surgical technique and make the dissection more difficult. Incontinence rates may therefore be higher;

Table 2.1 Patient risk factors for post-prostatectomy incontinence

Increase risk	Decrease risk
Obesity	Strong pelvic support
Older age	
Preoperative urinary incontinence	
Prior radiation therapy	

however, this is likely due to the surgery rather than the influence of advanced disease itself [31].

There are mixed findings on the influence of radiation therapy on incontinence in post-prostatectomy patients. Some groups report equivalent continence rates between patients who underwent adjuvant radiotherapy and those who did not [32]. However, patients who underwent a salvage prostatectomy following external beam radiotherapy have been shown to have significantly higher rates of incontinence [33], which some suggest may be related to external sphincter fibrosis secondary to radiation therapy. Table 2.1 lists patient risk factors for PPI.

While preoperative risk factors may be important in counseling patients prior to radical prostatectomy, they actually play little role the evaluation and management of PPI, with the exception of prior radiation therapy. Radiation can influence the type of evaluation done and the type of treatment recommended.

Influence of Surgical Techniques

The surgical technique utilized to perform a prostatectomy has been evaluated with respect to effect on rates of incontinence. Factors such as perineal vs. retropubic surgical approach [34–36], robot-assisted laparoscopic prostatectomy (RALP) vs. open retropubic [37–41], bladder neck preservation [42, 43], and nerve sparing [44–50] have been reported by some to improve continence, while others have found no difference. Table 2.1 summarizes some of the risk factors for PPI.

As with preoperative risk factors, surgical technique of radical prostatectomy plays little role the evaluation and management of PPI once it is established that the patient has incontinence and is seeking intervention.

Evaluation of Post-prostatectomy Incontinence

The approach to the initial evaluation of a patient with PPI is similar to that of any patient with incontinence, in that a careful evaluation of the quality and quantity of the incontinence should be determined, along with the effect on quality of life for the individual patient.

General Medical History

Age, as mentioned previously, should frame the clinician's understanding of the individual patient's problems and likelihood of long-term continence [51]. The time interval since RP should also be determined, given the time-dependent nature of return to continence (see Incidence).

Additional interventions for treatment of prostate cancer should also be determined. A history of radiation therapy, or current or future treatment of metastatic or locally recurrent disease may influence evaluation, timing, or type of treatment [51]. Prior surgeries, especially involving the pelvis, and radiation therapy for purposes other than treatment of prostate cancer should be determined. The current stage and status of prostate cancer should be elicited.

Other medical conditions should be evaluated. For example, a neurogenic bladder can result from a history of trauma or surgery, and should be on the differential, if present [4].

Medications should be reviewed. Certain medications act directly on the GU tract and affect continence, for example alpha-adrenergic blockers can decrease urethral tone and can contribute to urinary incontinence, and anticholinergics may inhibit detrusor contractility. Other medications may indirectly contribute to UI, such as angiotensin-converting enzymes that can cause a chronic cough (exacerbation of SUI) and diuretics that increase voided volumes,

which can exacerbate symptoms of urgency and frequency [4].

Finally, an evaluation of the patient's overall health and performance status is important when considering therapy. Elderly patients are more likely to be on multiple medications, and so careful assessment of potential drug interactions is important when initiating new drug therapy aimed to treat UI. In addition, anticholinergic medications can have significant effects on cognition in the elderly patient, and decision to treat with this medication should be made based on a risk–benefit assessment. There are limited studies evaluating the success or complication rates following operative intervention, however it is generally recommended to ensure that the benefit outweighs any operative risk and to ensure patients have sufficient performance status to recover well from a surgical intervention [4]. For an artificial urinary sphincter (AUS), for example, a patient must have sufficient hand dexterity and strength to use the device.

The evaluation of a patient with post-prostatectomy incontinence should begin with an assessment of the patient's general medical history. This includes age, time interval since prostatectomy, additional prior interventions for treatment of prostate cancer, other medical problems, and medication history. Importantly, the patient's performance status and overall health should frame clinician counseling on intervention options.

Characterization of Incontinence and Other Lower Urinary Tract Symptoms

Characterization of the quantity and type of the UI and the circumstances under which it occurs are important to help elucidate the cause and the severity of the symptoms.

It is important to determine whether the patient considers the incontinence to be stress-related (involuntary loss of urine with activity, cough, or other event that increases intra-abdominal pressure) urgency-related (involuntary loss of associated with urgency), or a combination of both [52]. If both are present it is important to try to determine which is more predominant and more bothersome. Sometimes patients are unable to express if urine loss is caused by activity or urgency. Incontinence can be insensible (occurring without stress or urgency) or may require more pointed questions as to when incontinence occurs (exactly what the patient is doing during incontinence episodes). In addition, a gravitational component to UI can increase suspicion for sphincteric incompetence as the underlying cause if UI worsens with sitting to standing or while standing, as compared to UI while lying down. Focusing on specific activities that cause or increase incontinence can be especially helpful for the patient with rare UI, where it is difficult to characterize the incontinence in great detail. A study by Mungovan et al. found that the activities that most commonly provoke urinary leakage in post-prostatectomy patients were walking at a comfortable speed and drinking fluids while seated [53]. Identifying the precipitating factors in an individual patient can help the clinician determine the type of incontinence present, and ultimately the intervention that would be most beneficial. Also, some patients will complain that incontinence worsens towards the late afternoon or evening hours. When not associated with urgency, this is thought to occur as a result of "sphincter fatigue" in patients with underlying sphincteric dysfunction. Some patients will experience incontinence due to sexual arousal or orgasm. We believe this is mostly due to sphincteric insufficiency. It can be difficult to manage when it is the only time that a man experiences incontinence.

It is also very important to determine the severity of the incontinence. This is commonly done on an objective basis by assessing pad usage (see below). For patients with more severe incontinence, we find it useful to ask if they are able to voluntarily void at all when they are active. If the answer is no, it is usually a sign of severe sphincteric insufficiency.

With respect to other LUTS, we find it helpful to determine the presence of any overactive bladder symptoms (urinary frequency and urgency not related to incontinence) and nocturia. This knowledge can help to set reasonable expectations from treatment. Also the force of the urinary stream and subjective voiding pattern can be helpful to know. When decreased or abnormal, it may raise the suspicion of a stricture. However, some men who are totally incontinent will report very poor stream because they actually never void significant amounts. For these patients, it can be useful to ask about voiding when they get up from bed with a relatively "full" bladder.

Overall, the patient's degree of bother related to urinary incontinence should be determined, as this will ultimately influence the patient's decision on pursuing further treatment or continuing conservative management. Relevant questions pertaining to the patient's history are summarized in Table 2.2.

Characterization of the subjective type and degree of incontinence as well as any other LUTS is important as it may prompt further testing prior to intervention and can sometimes have a profound effect of the type of treatment offered.

Physical Exam

The physical examination in the man with PPI should include several facets. The abdominal exam should include evaluation of the surgical scar. Palpation of the bladder in the lower abdomen should be performed to rule out a distended bladder to point towards an obstructive process. A digital rectal examination (DRE) will aid in assessment of rectal tone to help evaluate for neurologic factors, as well as a neurological examination of the perineum and lower extremities [4]. The most important part of the exam is the evaluation of the perineum, genitalia and stress testing for incontinence. A full genital examination should be performed. The quality if the skin of the scrotum and perineum should be evaluated. The patient should be observed for gravitational incontinence and then asked to cough or bear down to evaluate for stress urinary incontinence [4]. If the patient admits it incontinence with

Table 2.2 Patient history questions

Patient characteristics
Age
Weight
Mobility and activity?
Surgical characteristics
Time since surgery
Type of surgery
Interventions following surgery (medical or surgical)
Prior abdominal or pelvic surgery
Radiation therapy
Medical history
Other medical problems?
Neurologic problems?
Medication list?
Constipation or fecal incontinence?
Characteristics of controlled voiding
Force of stream
Emptying bladder to completion
Split stream
Characteristics of incontinence
Stress and/or urgency
Awareness of leakage (insensible)
Gravitational
Frequency of leakage
Degree or volume of leakage (number, size, wetness of pads)
Precipitating events or activities
Pattern of incontinence (day versus night)
Degree of bother

certain maneuvers (e.g., bending) he should be asked to perform such maneuvers especially if stress incontinence is not otherwise demonstrated. If the patient is wearing a protective pad, the wetness and size of the pad can be assessed during the physical exam. Though rare, meatal stenosis and phimosis can occur after prostatectomy, and should be ruled out as a cause of obstruction on examination [51].

The physical exam should include an abdominal exam and a full genital exam. In addition, assessment for stress urinary incontinence, including provocative maneuvers that cause incontinence elicited from the patient history, should be performed.

Voiding Diaries and Questionnaires

A voiding and intake diary (bladder diary) is an objective way for patients to describe both frequency and volume of voids, and is designed to include a description of episodes of urinary leakage, fluid intake, and the presence and degree of urgency associated with leakage over a 3–7 day period [4]. The use of bladder diaries in the context of PPI is primarily of use when patients have significant urge UI, and are an inexpensive way to objectify the symptoms for the clinician to interpret [54]. It provides information on the patient's voiding patterns and can shed light on bladder capacity. It can also identify excessive fluid intake [29]. Bladder diaries can be used to monitor changes in urge-related incontinence symptoms, whether over time or following an intervention, and for this reason are useful for measuring outcome [55].

Drawbacks to the use of diaries include patient difficulty in completing them accurately and in a timely manner, which increases as the number of days recorded increase. Also, urinary leakage that occurs less than once daily will have a limited ability to be represented. The Fifth International Consultation on Incontinence (ICUD) provided recommendations in their *Incontinence* text in 2013 in which they give a grade C recommendation (based on expert opinion) for the use of bladder diaries in the initial evaluation of patients with PPI to help communicate voiding patterns [4].

Questionnaires are another useful tool to objectively measure symptoms and their influence on quality of life, and are a more commonly utilized tool in patients with PPI. There are many available questionnaires that can be focused on symptoms, measures of patient-reported outcomes, or influence on quality of life. Patients with obstructive symptoms can have their symptoms characterized by questionnaires such as the American Urological Association score for BPH (AUA-7) [56], and the International Prostate Symptom Score (IPSS) [57]. Patients with urgency symptoms can be better assessed with the International Consultation on Incontinence Modular Questionnaire (ICIQ) [58]. The European Association of Urology published guidelines on management of urinary incontinence in 2014 where they provided a grade B recommendation (based on well-conducted clinical nonrandomized trials) on the use of questionnaires as a way to provide a standardized assessment of voiding symptoms [55].

For the patient with PPI, voiding and intake diaries and questionnaires are not an essential part of the evaluation in routine clinical practice for all patients. Diaries are most useful when there are complaints of overactive bladder symptoms, nocturia or nocturnal enuresis as a predominant complaint (especially if daytime incontinence is minimal). Diaries may also be useful in cases where excessive fluid intake is suspected. Questionnaires are most beneficial in the research setting, but can be useful when trying to differentiate stress for urgency incontinence in cases where direct questioning is less conclusive (e.g., the MESA questionnaire)[59].

Pad Usage and Pad Tests

Determining the number of pads a patient with PPI requires has been shown to affect patient's perception of degree of severity of incontinence. Fowlers et al. found that patients who wore pads were more likely to report urinary leakage as a medium or big problem than those who did not require pads but still reported urinary leakage [23]. The number of pads required also influences patient perception of continence. Sacco et al. showed that patients requiring one pad daily consider themselves continent and have good perception of health-related QoL (HRQoL), while requirement of two or pads daily had worse HRQoL outcomes, and patients were less likely to consider themselves continent [60].

Pad tests are often used to help evaluate the relationship between the patient's sensation of urinary leakage and the actual volume of urine leaked. Several studies have shown that quantifying incontinence by pad weights or pad number can predict outcomes of certain interventions [4].

We believe that a 24-h pad test is the gold standard objective measurement of PPI. The number of pads is not a perfect measure of leakage, as some patients will tolerate a saturated pad prior to changing, while others may change pads frequently with even mild leakage. In addition, there is variability in the size and type of pad [4]. Tsui et al. showed that the severity of incontinence was not related to the number of pads used, but better correlated to the pad weight, and recommends that pad weight be used rather than pad count alone [61]. However, there is evidence that a pad test may not be absolutely necessary to quantify the degree incontinence, provided that patients can accurately express the size, number and wetness of the pads that they use. In a prospective study conducted by the SUFU foundation, patient perception of number of pads required on a daily basis correlated well with actual number of pads collected during pad testing over a 24-h period. When patients were asked, "to what extent does urine loss affect your quality of life?" with options not at all, small amount, moderate amount and significant amount, they were stratified into four groups which were shown to be different in the number of pads required [2]. The study concluded that a pad test might not necessary to accurately determine the severity of PPI, if carefully collected prospective information about incontinence is obtained.

We believe that an accurate assessment of the degree of incontinence is important before recommending certain interventions. The literature would support the premise that sling procedures are less effective in cases of severe incontinence. How one assesses the degree of incontinence will vary depending on the clinical scenario. If a patient wears multiple extra large pads/day (i.e., diapers) and admits that they are always wet to soaked, that may enough to conclude that incontinence is severe. Conversely if the patient is wearing one extra small or small pad per day incontinence is likely mild (or moderate at the worst). However the majority of patient fall between these two extremes. In such cases formal pad testing, or a least an accurate assessment of pad number, size and wetness is recommended.

Simple Diagnostic Studies

A urinalysis is generally recommended as an initial diagnostic study for patients with urinary incontinence to rule out an infectious cause, along with a urine culture [15]. In addition, older men are at risk of diseases of the bladder such as bladder cancer, carcinoma in situ, bladder stones, and urethral strictures, often presenting with overactive bladder symptoms, which can be reflected in hematuria or pyuria. Performing a urinalysis can help rule out some of these causes of UI [4]. The EAU provides a grade A recommendation (based on clinical studies of good quality) for routinely performing a urinalysis [55].

A post-void residual (PVR) helps assess for incomplete emptying and obstruction as a cause of voiding symptoms. The Canadian Urological Association (CUA) published guidelines on adult UI in 2012 and provides a grade A recommendation (based on clinical studies of good quality) to include a PVR as part of the routine assessment [62]. The American Urological Association also recommend in their guidelines on the surgical management of SUI, updated in 2009, to perform a PVR as an essential part of the patient evaluation [63]. There are not specific values associated with abnormal PVRs [54], however it provides the clinician an understanding of the patient's ability to empty their bladder, which can be related to symptoms. The ICUD recommends that a PVR of greater than 200 mL should be considered a sign of an obstructive urinary problem [4]. Uroflowmetry, similar to assessment of PVR, is useful in assessing for obstructive urinary patterns [15].

Routine assessment of bladder emptying is important in the evaluation of PPI. This is most easily accomplished by determination of a post void residual (or random check of bladder volume in a patient with severe incontinence who does not void). This is most commonly done by a bladder scan ultrasound. Uroflow is generally reserved for patients who complain of some emptying symptoms (incomplete emptying or slow stream).

Imaging for PPI

Differences on imaging have been shown to exist between patients with and without incontinence following a prostatectomy. These studies have been performed to help elucidate causes of PPI, rather than helping evaluate degree or outcomes of urinary incontinence. Tuygun et al. performed pelvic magnetic resonance imaging (MRI) on patients following prostatectomy and found that patients with PPI had a higher incidence of fibrosis, thereby concluding that fibrosis plays a key factor in the pathogenesis of PPI [64].

Paparel et al. studied the change in urethral length on preoperative and postoperative pelvic MRIs in patients undergoing radical prostatectomy and found that membranous urethral length loss was associated with incontinence, and recommend preservation of this length intraoperatively to help improve continence [65].

In clinical practice, imaging does not have a significant role in evaluating PPI and predicting treatment outcomes unless other pathologies are being excluded, for example fistulae or underlying cancerous processes [55]. The most common form of imaging is the voiding cystourethrogram done as part of videourodynamics. While this can provide a very accurate anatomic assessment of the lower urinary tract, it has not been found to be superior to standard urodynamics in a head to head trial.

Urodynamics

Urodynamic studies (UDS) remain the gold standard for diagnosing the type of incontinence in patients post-prostatectomy. However, it is not always a requirement to perform in the setting of PPI. Urodynamics can be used to diagnose bladder dysfunction such as detrusor overactivity or decreased compliance and the capacity of the bladder. It can also be used to determine the abdominal leak point pressure (ALPP), which, in men following a prostatectomy, is primarily related to sphincteric incompetence [4].

It is important to note that urodynamics may not serve to predict outcome following intervention, but serve to diagnose the type of incontinence present. Thiel et al. failed to find a urodynamic parameter that would identify those patients who failed artificial urinary sphincter (AUS) placement, with failure defined as requiring one pad or more following placement [66]. Similarly, ALPP may provide an "objective measure" of urethral resistance to an increase in abdominal pressure but fails to predict surgical outcomes [67]. Twiss et al. evaluated 29 patients with SUI following prostatectomy and found that ALPP on UDS failed to correlate with their degree of urinary incontinence, as determined by the 24-h pad test. They concluded that ALPP has limited clinical value in the setting of PPI management, and recommend focusing on the presence or absence of SUI and bladder dysfunction during urodynamics to guide management and diagnosis [20].

Symptoms alone are inferior to urodynamics for diagnostic purposes. Reis et al. evaluated patients with urinary incontinence following radical prostatectomy and compared their responses on the International Consultation on Incontinence Questionnaire-Short Form (ICIQ-UISF) to their findings on urodynamic studies (diagnoses included sphincteric incontinence alone, bladder dysfunction, and a combination of these two). They found that the diagnosis determined by urodynamics were not predicted by the ICIQ-UISF and concluded that urodynamic testing is required for determining the etiology of incontinence [22]. However the routine use of urodynamics has not been shown to result in better treatment outcomes for PPI. It is important to note that treating SUI symptoms in the presence of bladder dysfunction does not alter outcomes in PPI patients. Ballert and Nitti examined 72 PPI men with SUI, of which 30.6 % had concomitant detrusor overactivity, and found that preoperative detrusor overactivity did not result in worse postoperative outcomes. They caution, however, that these patients may require anticholinergic treatment postoperatively to improve symptoms [68]. Other

groups have found similar outcomes following placement of an AUS [69, 70].

There are some unique problems encountered in PPI patients when performing UDS. A bladder neck contracture/anastomotic structure can be narrow enough that even the small caliber urethral catheters used for UDS, 7-French, can be sufficient to occlude the urethra and limit the ability to measure VLPP. For patients where sphincteric incompetence is strongly suspected, but no leakage is noted, it is suggested that the study be repeated. Another problem may arise in patients with severe sphincteric insufficiency, where standing upright results in continuous leakage. Methods to help manage this incontinence during urodynamics are use of a penile clamp or having a patient lay supine during filling [71].

Urodynamics should be an option in patients who are considering advanced treatment of incontinence (either surgical intervention for stress incontinence or third line therapy for urgency incontinence). Urodynamics is not necessary or practical for patients who have had recent prostatectomy and are still in the recovery phase or for patients considering conservative or medical treatment of incontinence. While some routinely recommend urodynamics prior to a surgical intervention, the utility of this practice has not been proven to affect outcomes [15]. The AUA/SUFU Urodynamics Guideline states that "clinicians should perform repeat stress testing with the urethral catheter removed in patients suspected of having SUI who do not demonstrate this finding with the catheter in place during urodynamic testing" [72]. It is also known that in PPI the urethral catheter can cause obstruction due to the rigidity of the anastomotic area. For this reason we generally subscribe to the urodynamics protocol we published in 2005 for specific use in the post-prostatectomy male with urinary incontinence [71]. As per standard urodynamic protocol, a 7 Fr urethral catheter and a rectal catheter should be used, with pressure sensors to determine the detrusor pressure from their difference. It is recommended to initiate filling at a medium fill rate, starting at 50 mL/min but reduce to 30 mL/min in patients with a history of severe urgency incontinence or a known small functional bladder capacity. As mentioned previously, for patients with severe sphincteric incompetence, a penile clamp can be used to allow bladder filling in the standing position. We recommend filling to 150 mL and then performing straining maneuvers to assess for stress incontinence. If incontinence is detected, an abdominal leak point pressure (ALPP) can be determined. If no stress incontinence is demonstrated, filling is continued and Stress incontinence is assessed at various volumes (usually 50 mL intervals) until demonstrated. If stress incontinence is not demonstrated, it should be reassessed for without a catheter at a volume of at least 50 % of cystometric capacity. At capacity, a pressure-flow study is performed, as is the standard in urodynamics. Video fluoroscopy can be performed to evaluate both the bladder neck as well as the region of the anastomosis to assess for the presence of a narrowing or stricture. In these patients at risk for a scarred urethra, a urethral catheter can occlude the urethra and prevent diagnosis of sphincteric insufficiency (35 % of this study's population), and the ALPP may be falsely elevated [71]. For this reason, Huckabay et al. recommend a second fill phase to 50–70 % of bladder capacity on first fill phase, followed by removal of the catheter and reassess for stress incontinence (and ALPP if desired). A noninvasive uroflow can be obtained and a repeat video fluoroscopy. A urodynamic protocol for PPI evaluation is shown in Fig. 2.1.

Urodynamics can be helpful is assessing the patient with PPI. Controlled studies regarding the value of UDS in PPI have not been done. Practically speaking, clinicians should do UDS prior to advanced therapy if the information provided will help to guide treatment or patient counseling. UDS is also useful in cases when the clinician is not sure of the cause of the problem. Although there is no evidence-base literature to support or refute UDS in patients who have had radiation, at this time we would rec-ommend routine use in such patients who are considering surgical intervention. Finally we also believe that UDS is valuable in men who have PPI with incomplete bladder emptying, not caused by an obvious stricture.

Cystoscopy

In patients who have symptomatic decreased force of stream and incomplete emptying, cysto-urethroscopy should be performed to rule out abnormalities such as a urethral stricture or bladder neck contracture [15]. It should also be performed if other bladder abnormalities are suspected, such as diverticulum, bladder stones, and presence of staples in the bladder [51]. It is also recommended that cystourethroscopy be performed prior to any surgical intervention, to evaluate for any urethral scarring and to evaluate the status of the bladder [15].

Cystourethroscopy should be preformed routinely before surgical intervention such as artificial urinary sphincter or sling procedure to evaluate the urethra, anastomosis and bladder.

Summary

Post-prostatectomy incontinence most often primarily due to sphincteric incompetence related to the surgical intervention, though bladder dysfunction can be present in isolation or in combination with stress incontinence. An understanding of the risk factors for PPI, including older age and obesity, should be evaluated, and an understanding of the different risks of urinary incontinence can help risk-stratify patients for long term voiding dysfunction. The complexity of the evaluation of PPI is determined by the degree of bother to the patient and his willingness to proceed with treatment. A detailed history and physical (including the use of questionnaires and bladder diaries when indicated) can provide important information in guiding diagnosis of the

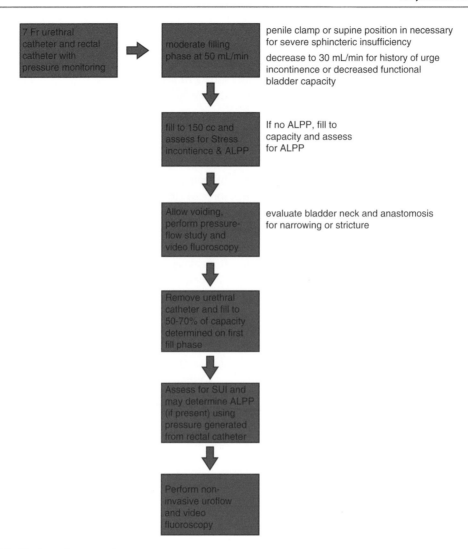

Fig. 2.1 Urodynamics protocol

type of incontinence. An accurate assessment of the degree (quantity) of incontinence is important and this can be aided by pad testing or careful questioning. Imaging has low utility in diagnosis of PPI, unless combined with urodynamics (videourodynamics). Cystourethroscopy has utility in select cases, and is recommended prior to surgical intervention for evaluation of the urethra, anastomosis and bladder. Urodynamics may also be performed prior to surgical intervention if it will influence treatment and/or counseling. This helps guide appropriate intervention and management. A pathway for initial evaluation of PPI Patients is shown in Fig. 2.2.

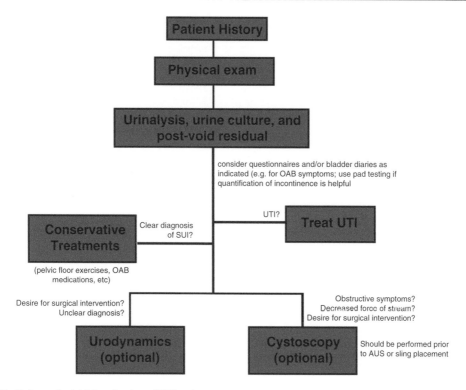

Fig. 2.2 Pathway for initial evaluation of PPI patients

References

1. Ficazzola MA, Nitti VW. The etiology of post-radical prostatectomy incontinence and correlation of symptoms with urodynamic findings. J Urol. 1998;160(4): 1317–20.
2. Nitti VW, Mourtzinos A, Brucker BM. SUFU Pad Test Study Group. Correlation of patient perception of pad use with objective degree of incontinence measured by pad test in men with post-prostatectomy incontinence: the SUFU Pad Test Study. J Urol. 2014;192(3):836–42.
3. Kao TC, Cruess DF, Garner D, et al. Multicenter patient self-reporting questionnaire on impotence, incontinence and stricture after radical prostatectomy. J Urol. 2000;163:858.
4. Abrams P, Cardozo L, Khoury S, Wein A. Incontinence. 5th ed. Paris, France: European Association of Urology - International Consultation on Incontinence; 2013.
5. Moinzadeh A, Shunaigat AN, Libertino JA. Urinary incontinence after radical retropubic prostatectomy: the outcome of a surgical technique. BJU Int. 2003;92:355.
6. Walsh PC, Marschke P, Ricker D, Burnett AL. Patient- reported urinary continence and sexual function after anatomic radical prostatectomy. Urology. 2000;55:58.
7. Kumar A, Nitti VW. Contemporary incidence of post-prostatectomy incontinence and impact on health-related quality of life. Curr Bladder Dysfunct Rep. 2010;5:135–41.
8. Penson DF, McLerran D, Feng Z, et al. 5-year urinary and sexual outcomes after radical prostatectomy: results from the prostate cancer outcomes study. J Urol. 2005;173:1701.
9. Goluboff ET, Saidi JA, Mazer S, et al. Urinary continence after radical prostatectomy: the Columbia experience. J Urol. 1998;159:1276.
10. Smither AR, Guralnick ML, Davis NB, See WA. Quantifying the natural history of post-radical prostatectomy incontinence using objective pad test data. BMC Urol. 2007;7:2.
11. Vickers AJ, Kent M, Mulhall J, Sandhu J. Counseling the post-radical prostatectomy patients about functional recovery: high predictiveness of current status. Urology. 2014;84(1):158–63.
12. Schneider T, Sperling H, Rossi R, Schmidt S, Rübben H. Do early injections of bulking agents following

radical prostatectomy improve early continence? World J Urol. 2005;23(5):338–42.

13. Jones JS, Vasavada SP, Abdelmalak JB. Sling may hasten return of continence after radical prostatectomy. Urology. 2005;65(6):1163–7.

14. Gosling JA, Dixon JS, Critchley HO, Thompson SA. A comparative study of the human external sphincter and periurethral levator ani muscles. Br J Urol. 1981;53:35–41.

15. Wein AJ, Kavoussi LR, Novick AC, Partin AW, Peters CA. Campbell-walsh urology. 10th ed. Philadelphia, PA: Elsevier Saunders; 2012.

16. Groutz A, Blaivas JG, Chaikin DC, et al. The pathophysiology of post-radical prostatectomy incontinence: a clinical and video urodynamic study. J Urol. 2000;163(6):1767–70.

17. Gudziak MR, McGuire EJ, Gormley EA. Urodynamic assessment of urethral sphincter function in postprostatectomy incontinence. J Urol. 1996;156(3):1131–4.

18. Desautel MG, Kapoor R, Badlani GH. Sphincteric incontinence: the primary cause of post-prostatectomy incontinence in patients with prostate cancer. Neurourol Urodyn. 1997;16(3):153–60.

19. Winters JC, Appell RA, Rackley RR. Urodynamic findings in postprostatectomy incontinence. Neurourol Urodyn. 1998;17(5):493–8.

20. Twiss C, Fleischmann N, Nitti VW. Correlation of abdominal leak point pressure with objective incontinence severity in men with post-radical prostatectomy stress incontinence. Neurourol Urodyn. 2005;24(3):207–10.

21. Giannantoni A, Mearini E, Di Stasi SM, et al. Assessment of bladder and urethral sphincter function before and after radical retropubic prostatectomy. J Urol. 2004;171(4):1563–6.

22. Reis RB, Cologna AJ, Machado RD, et al. Lack of association between the ICIQ-SF questionnaire and the urodynamic diagnosis in men with post radical prostatectomy incontinence. Acta Cir Bras. 2013;28 Suppl 1:37–42.

23. Fowler Jr FJ, Barry MJ, Lu-Yao G, Wasson J, Roman A, Wennberg J. Effect of radical prostatectomy for prostate cancer on patient quality of life: results from a Medicare survey. Urology. 1995;45(6):1007–13.

24. Collado SA, Rubio-Briones J, Pyol Payas M, Iborra Juan I, Ramon-Borja JC, Solsona NE. Postprostatectomy established stress urinary incontinence treated with duloxetine. Urology. 2011;78:261–6.

25. Wallerstedt A, Carlsson S, Steineck G, et al. Patient and tumour-related factors for prediction of urinary incontinence after radical prostatectomy. Scand J Urol. 2013;47(4):272–81.

26. Kim SC, Song C, Kim W, et al. Factors determining functional outcomes after radical prostatectomy: robot-assisted versus retropubic. Eur Urol. 2011;60(3):413–9.

27. Novara G, Ficarra V, D'elia C, et al. Evaluating urinary continence and preoperative predictors of urinary continence after robot assisted laparoscopic radical prostatectomy. J Urol. 2010;184(3):1028–33.

28. Catalona WJ, Carvalhal GF, Mager DE, Smith DS. Potency, continence and complication rates in 1,870 consecutive radical retropubic prostatectomies. J Urol. 1999;162(2):433–8.

29. Song C, Doo CK, Hong JH, Choo MS, Kim CS, Ahn H. Relationship between the integrity of the pelvic floor muscles and early recovery of continence after radical prostatectomy. J Urol. 2007;178(1):208–11.

30. Xu T, Wang X, Xia L, et al. robot-assisted prostatectomy in obese patients: how influential is obesity on operative outcomes? J Endourol. 2015;29:198–208.

31. Zincke H, Oesterling JE, Blute ML, et al. Long-term (15 years) results after radical prostatectomy for clinically localized (stage T2c or lower) prostate cancer. J Urol. 1994;152(5 Pt. 2):1850–7.

32. Petrovich Z, Lieskovsky G, Langholz B, et al. Comparison of outcomes of radical prostatectomy with and without adjuvant pelvic irradiation in patients with pathologic stage C (T3N0) adenocarcinoma of the prostate. Am J Clin Oncol. 1999;22(4):323–31.

33. Nguyen PL, D'Amico AV, Lee AK, Suh WW. Patient selection, cancer control, and complications after salvage local therapy for postradiation prostate-specific antigen failure: a systematic review of the literature. Cancer. 2007;110(7):1417–28.

34. Weldon VE, Tavel FR, Neuwirth H. Continence, potency and morbidity after radical perineal prostatectomy. J Urol. 1997;158:1470.

35. Gray M, Petroni GR, Theodorescu D. Urinary function after radical prostatectomy: a comparison of the retropubic and perineal approaches. Urology. 1999;53:881.

36. Sullivan LD, Weir MJ, Kinahan JF, Taylor DL. A comparison of the relative merits of radical perineal and radical retropubic prostatectomy. BJU Int. 2000;85(1):95–100.

37. Froehner M, Koch R, Leike S, Novotny V, Twelker L, Wirth MP. Urinary tract-related quality of life after radical prostatectomy: open retropubic versus robot-assisted laparoscopic approach. Urol Int. 2013;90(1):36–40.

38. Geraerts I, Van Poppel H, Devoogdt N, Van Cleynenbreugel B, Joniau S, Van Kampen M. Prospective evaluation of urinary incontinence, voiding symptoms and quality of life after open and robot-assisted radical prostatectomy. BJU Int. 2013;112(7):936–43.

39. Rocco B, Matei DV, Melegari S, et al. Robotic vs open prostatectomy in a laparoscopically naive centre: a matched-pair analysis. BJU Int. 2009;104:991–5.

40. Di Pierro GB, Baumeister P, Stucki P, Beatrice J, Danuser H, Mattei A. A prospective trial comparing

consecutive series of open retropubic and robot-assisted laparoscopic radical prostatectomy in a centre with a limited caseload. Eur Urol. 2011;59:1–6.

41. Krambeck AE, DiMarco DS, Rangel LJ, et al. Radical prostatectomy for prostatic adenocarcinoma: a matched comparison of open retropubic and robot-assisted techniques. BJU Int. 2009;103:448–53.

42. Srougi M, Nesrallah LJ, Kauffmann JR, Nesrallah A, Leite KR. Urinary continence and pathological outcome after bladder neck preservation during radical retropubic prostatectomy: a randomized prospective trial. J Urol. 2001;165:815.

43. Poon M, Ruckle H, Bamshad DBR, Rsai C, Webster R, Lui P. Radical retropubic prostatectomy: bladder neck preservation versus reconstruction. J Urol. 2000;163:194.

44. Burkhard FC, Kessler TM, Fleischmann A, et al. Nerve sparing open radical retropubic prostatectomy-does it have an impact on urinary continence? J Urol. 2006;179:189–95.

45. Nandipati KC, Raina R, Agarwal A, Zippe CD. Nerve-sparing surgery significantly affects long-term continence after radical prostatectomy. Urology. 2007;70:1127–30.

46. Choi WW, Freire MP, Soukup JR, et al. Nerve-sparing technique and urinary control after robot-assisted laparoscopic prostatectomy. World J Urol. 2011; 29:21–7.

47. Srivastava A, Chopra S, Pham A, et al. Effect of a risk-stratified grade of nerve-sparing technique on early return of continence after robot-assisted laparoscopic radical prostatectomy. Eur Urol. 2013;63: 38–44.

48. Marien TP, Lepor H. Does a nerve-sparing technique or potency affect continence after open radical retropubic prostatectomy? BJU Int. 2008;102:1581–4.

49. Tzou DT, Dalkin BL, Christopher BA, Cui H. The failure of a nerve sparing template to improve urinary continence after radical prostatectomy: attention to study design. Urol Oncol. 2009;27:358–62.

50. Peterson AC, Chen Y. Patient reported incontinence after radical prostatectomy is more common than expected and not associated with the nerve sparing technique: results from the Center for Prostate Disease Research (CPDR) Database. Neurourol Urodyn. 2012;31:60–3.

51. Radomski SB. Practical evaluation of post-prostatectomy incontinence. Can Urol Assoc J. 2013;7(9–10 Suppl 4):S186–8.

52. Abrams P, Cardozo L, Fall M, et al. The standardization of terminology of lower urinary tract function: report from the Standardization Sub-committee of the International Continence Society. Neurourol Urodyn. 2002;21:167–78.

53. Mungovan SF, Huijbers BP, Hirschhorn AD, Patel MI. What makes men leak? An investigation of objective and self-report measures of urinary incontinence early after radical prostatectomy. Neurourol Urodyn. 2014. doi:10.1002/nau.22701.

54. Flynn BJ, Webster GD. Evaluation and surgical management of intrinsic sphincter deficiency after radical prostatectomy. Rev Urol. 2004;6(4):180–6.

55. Lucas MG, Bedretdinova D, Bosch JLHR et al. EAU Guidelines on urinary incontinence. Eur Assoc Urol 2014, update April 2014

56. Svatek R, Roche V, Thornberg J, Zimmern P. Normative values for the American Urological Association Symptom Index (AUA-7) and short form Urogenital Distress Inventory (UDI-6) in patients 65 and older presenting for non-urological care. Neurourol Urodyn. 2005;24(7):606–10.

57. Bayoud Y, de la Taille A, Ouzzane A, et al. International Prostate Symptom Score is a predictive factor of lower urinary tract symptoms after radical prostatectomy. Int J Urol. 2015;22:283–7.

58. Abrams P, Avery K, Gardener N, Donovan J, ICIQ Advisory Board. The International Consultation on Incontinence Modular Questionnaire: www.iciq.net. J Urol. 2006;175(3 Pt 1):1063–6.

59. Ogunyemi TO, Siadat MR, Arslanturk S, Killinger KA, Diokno AC. Novel application of statistical methods to identify new urinary incontinence risk factors. Adv Urol. 2012;2012:p1–8.

60. Sacco E, Prayer-Galetti T, Pinto F, et al. Urinary incontinence after radical prostatectomy: incidence by definition, risk factors, and temporal trend in a large series with a long-term follow-up. BJU Int. 2006;97:1234–41.

61. Tsui JF, Shah MB, Weinberger JM, et al. Pad count is a poor measure of the severity of urinary incontinence. J Urol. 2013;190(5):1787–90.

62. Bettez M, Tu LM, Carlson K, et al. CUA Guideline 2012 Update: guidelines for Adult Urinary Incontinence Collaborative Consensus Document for the Canadian Urological Association. Can Urol Assoc J. 2012;6(5):354–63.

63. Dmochowski RR, Blaivas JM, Gormley EA, et al. Update of AUA guideline on the surgical management of female stress urinary incontinence. J Urol. 2010;183(5):1906–14.

64. Tuygun C, Imamoglu A, Keyik B, Alisir I, Yorubulut M. Significance of fibrosis around and/or at external urinary sphincter on pelvic magnetic resonance imaging in patients with postprostatectomy incontinence. Urology. 2006;68(6):1308–12.

65. Paparel P, Akin O, Sandhu JS, et al. Recovery of urinary continence after radical prostatectomy: association with urethral length and urethral fibrosis measured by preoperative and postoperative endorectal magnetic resonance imaging. Eur Urol. 2009;55(3):629–37.

66. Thiel DD, Young PR, Broderick GA, et al. Do clinical or urodynamic parameters predict artificial urinary sphincter outcome in post-radical prostatectomy incontinence? Urology. 2007;69(2):315–9.

67. Soljanik I, Becker AJ, Stief CG, Gozzi C, Bauer RM. Urodynamic parameters after retrourethral transobturator male sling and their influence on outcome. Urology. 2011;78(3):708–12.

68. Ballert KN, Nitti VW. Association between detrusor overactivity and postoperative outcomes in patients undergoing male bone anchored perineal sling. J Urol. 2010;183(2):641–5.
69. Pérez LM, Webster GD. Successful outcome of artificial urinary sphincters in men with post-prostatectomy urinary incontinence despite adverse implantation features. J Urol. 1992;148(4): 1166–70.
70. Lai HH, Hsu EI, Boone TB. Urodynamic testing in evaluation of postradical prostatectomy incontinence before artificial urinary sphincter implantation. Urology. 2009;73(6):1264–9.
71. Huckabay C, Twiss C, Berger A, Nitti VW. A urodynamics protocol to optimally assess men with post-prostatectomy incontinence. Neurourol Urodyn. 2005;24(7):622–6.
72. Gormley EA, Lightner DJ, Burgio KL et al. Diagnosis and treatment of overactive bladder (non-neurogenic) in adults: AUA/SUFU guideline 2014 update. The American Urological Association Education and Research, Inc. 2014 Linthicum, Maryland.

Urinary Incontinence: Conservative and Medical Management and Injectable Therapy

3

Hajar I. Ayoub and Ouida Lenaine Westney

Introduction

The reported percentage of patients experiencing any leakage at 6 months post radical prostatectomy has ranged widely from 8 to 87 [1]. A significant amount of resolution occurs between the 6 and 12 month time period. However, the question remains what the best strategy is for accelerating the process to continence. Meanwhile, the patient will require assistance in managing the ongoing leakage in a manner that is comfortable, anxiety reducing and cost efficient [2].

Conservative Therapy

Absorbent Products: Liners, Guards, Briefs, Underwear

Strategies for the management of post prostatectomy urinary incontinence after catheter removal are influenced in the long-term by the volume of incontinence. Regardless, the majority of patients will start with absorbent pads with adjustments in type based on the severity of leakage [3]. Though not exhaustive, Table 3.1 details some of the currently commercially available types of male incontinence protection by size and absorbent capability. In general, milder incontinence is managed satisfactorily with shields or lower density guards while severe incontinence requires brief or underwear with or without inserts to prevent accidents. As the requirement for absorbent capacity increases, the stability of the system must be enhanced to tolerate more fluid (Figs. 3.1, 3.2, 3.3, and 3.4). The brief and underwear configurations also are available in a variety of sizes to accommodate differing body habitus. From a cost perspective, briefs and underwear systems have been demonstrated to be more effective than pads [4]. Thus, the patient should be advised along these lines if they wish to continue wearing pads as their primary mechanism for urinary containment.

In the individual patient, absorbent products alone may constitute a long-term management strategy. However, it has been demonstrated that the use of even one pad per day is a source of bother and decreased patient satisfaction [5]. Additionally, the use of pads may be associated with skin irritation and dermatitis, especially in the intertriginous areas. In those who need to change their pad or garment more than several pads per day, financial considerations may influence the ability to change pads in a timely fashion. Therefore, it is important to ensure that the patient is utilizing the most effective product based on their degree of incontinence.

H.I. Ayoub, M.D. • O.L. Westney, M.D. (✉)
Department of Urology, The University of Texas MD Anderson Cancer Center, Houston, TX, USA
e-mail: owestney@mdanderson.org

© Springer International Publishing Switzerland 2016
J.S. Sandhu (ed.), *Urinary Dysfunction in Prostate Cancer*, DOI 10.1007/978-3-319-23817-3_3

Table 3.1 Male absorbent protection by incontinence severity

	Mild	Moderate	Severe
Shields	Depend® Shields for Men Prevail® Belted Shields		
Guards	TENA® MEN™ Protective Guards—Level 1 Prevail® Male Guards	TENA® MEN™ Protective Guards—Level 2 Depend® Guards for Men	TENA® MEN™ Protective Guards—Level 3
Underwear		Prevail® Boxers for Men Prevail® Per-fit® Underwear	TENA® MEN™ Protective Underwear (Super Plus, (Plus and Extra) Absorbency Depend® for Men Underwear With FIT-FLEX™ Protection
Briefs			TENA® Classic Briefs Depend® Real Fit® Briefs for Men
Pad/pants systems			TENA® Day (Light, Regular, Plus) and Night Super Pads Prevail® Pant Liners

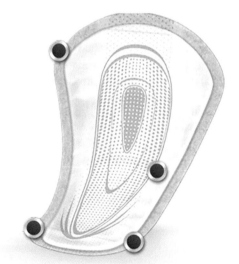

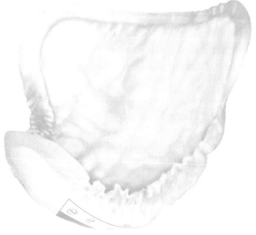

Fig. 3.2 Male guard

Fig. 3.1 Male shield

Occlusive Therapy (Penile Clamps)

Occlusive devices may function as a stand-alone therapy for incontinence or as an adjunct to absorbent products. Combination therapy between the two types of devices decreases the number of pads required during active periods with a resultant decrease in incontinence products expenditure. Penile clamps, while somewhat unsophisticated, are very effective when utilized properly. Satisfaction with this device is generally dependent on the ability to tolerate the penile

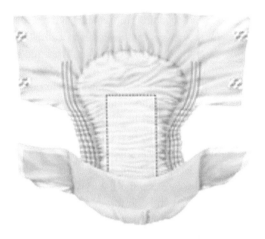

Fig. 3.3 Male brief type garment (diaper configuration)

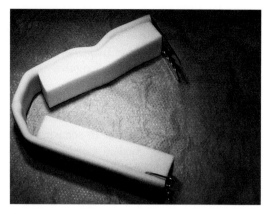

Fig. 3.5 Cunningham penile clamp

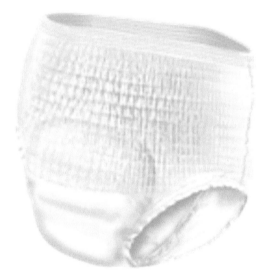

Fig. 3.4 Male absorbency underwear garment

compression in the mid-shaft. One of the most commonly used products of this type is the Cunningham clamp (Fig. 3.5). The clamp is available in three sizes (juvenile, regular, and large) corresponding to shaft length. Patients must be instructed to release the clamp every 2 h to allow for circulation regardless of whether it coincides with a void attempt. Additionally, the clamp should not be left on the phallus overnight due to the risks of constant pressure. Mechanical compression devices are not suitable for patients with memory deficits, poor manual dexterity,

impaired sensation or a significant component of overactive bladder.

Clamp type devices are available in three general styles: (1) Padded Straight, (2) Circular, and (3) Pouch (Table 3.2). The pouch type (Acticuf®) is distinguished by the addition of an absorbent pouch attached to a spring action clamp (Fig. 3.6a, b). One disadvantage of this model is the inability to customize the degree of compression. Additionally, device usage is defined by the limits of the pouch absorbency. Regardless, it is a viable option for patients with intermittent, low volume leakage.

Though simple in concept, penile clamps are not complication free even in appropriately selected patients. Moore et al. compared the Cunningham clamp, U-Tex adjustable strap, and the C3 clamp. While the Cunningham clamp was most successful in decreasing urine loss, it was associated with decreased penile Doppler flow and more discomfort [6]. In general, there are no predictors for which patients will find the clamps to be an indispensable tool versus those who describe it as "weapon of torture." Therefore, it should be suggested to all incontinent patients who do not have a contraindication.

Catheters (Condom, Urethral and Suprapubic)

Patients with severe or total incontinence may resort to a catheter and drainage system as the best method to obtain complete control of urinary incontinence. This form of management is advantageous when the number or frequency of absorbent product changes is disruptive and/or financially prohibitive.

Condom type catheters or urinary sheaths are an effective method of urinary containment for men with severe incontinence. In comparison to compressive devices, condom catheter systems are acceptable for patients with any degree of urge incontinence. Theoretically, this approach would also be superior to urethral catheterization due to the avoidance of mechanical bladder irritation. However, this management is unsuitable for patients with a retractile phallus, skin excoriation, concomitant urethral stricture, poor manual dexterity, or a large glans/narrow phallus configuration [7]. In the appropriate patient, external catheters have been demonstrated to be superior

to absorbent products in patient satisfaction. However, the success of a condom catheter is wholly dependent on proper sizing. The condom or sheath varies based on the material (latex or silicone), length of adhesive surface, circumference and overall length [8]. Ideally, the assistance of a continence nurse is highly desirable to ensure that the patient uses the best type for his anatomy. Alternatively, catheter suppliers will generally forward patients an assortment of condom catheters to allow for selection of the style that maintains an adherent and comfortable fit.

Urethral Catheter Drainage is a decision of last resort in a patient who is unsuitable for alternative management. The need for urethral catheterization may also reflect the presence of an unstable bladder neck due to an intractable stricture. Suprapubic catheter drainage is not an answer for the patient with severe incontinence secondary to an open bladder neck due to continued urethral leakage.

Table 3.2 Mechanical penile compression devices

	Name	Manufacturer
Padded clamp	Cunningham Clamp	BARD
	Dribble Stop	DribbleStop
	Squeezer Klip	Life Control
Circular	J Clamp	Jackson Medical Products
	C3	Personal Medical Corporation
	Uriclak	Uriclak
	U-Tex	
Pouch	Acticuf	GT Urological

Behavioral Therapy (Pelvic Floor Muscle Exercises, Biofeedback, Pelvic Floor Stimulation, and Lifestyle Adjustments)

Pelvic Floor Muscle Therapy (PFMT)

PFMT is a generic label for exercises meant to strengthen the pelvic floor musculature with resultant decreased leakage during periods of

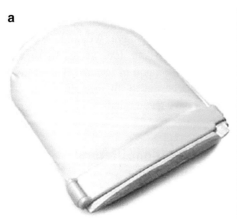
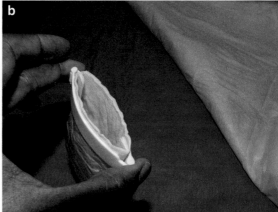

Fig. 3.6 (**a**) Acticuf penile clamp with pouch. (**b**) Open acticuf

increased intra-abdominal pressure combined with a reflex inhibitory effect on the detrusor body. Levels of instruction may range from simple verbal description to supervised physical therapy sessions. Assessment of the quality and strength of the contractions can arise from direct physical examination or via the use of biofeedback equipment. Pelvic floor muscle therapy programs are highly variable depending on the involvement of a therapist, specific pelvic floor contraction instructions, utilization of biofeedback, time of initiation, and number of exercises (contractions) prescribed per session and daily. A direct comparative analysis of the literature in this area has been complicated by varying exercise protocols and heterogeneous endpoints [9–11].

Basic PFMT initiates with verbal and written instruction in the outpatient setting combined with specific details regarding the number of contractions to be performed daily. While formal PFMT session with a licensed physiotherapist is an asset, it may not be critical to long-term continence outcomes. Moore et al. demonstrated equivalent continence outcomes in patients randomized to a formal PFMT session versus written/verbal instructions with phone support [10]. In this particular study, the self-directed program consisted of 10–12 pelvic floor muscle (PFM) exercises three times per day. In our clinical setting, the patients are given written and verbal instructions to perform 4–5 sets of 15 PFM's per day. Physical confirmation via digital examination while performing an exercise or consultation with a physiotherapist is reserved for patients with difficulty consistently recruiting the correct muscles and/or poorly sustained contractions.

Initiation of PFMT

There have been several randomized control trials (RCTs) evaluating the utility of starting PFMT prior to prostatectomy with the goal of improving time to continence and overall dry rates [12–15]. As previously stated, comparison of studies is difficult due to heterogeneity in patient populations, therapeutic protocols and endpoints. Differences in radical prostatectomy technique (open, robotic assisted, and laparoscopic assisted) introduce another source of incongruity between trials. Meta-analysis of RCTs preoperative and postoperative PFMT to postoperative PFMT only has failed to demonstrate a difference in continence between the two groups at 1-month, 3-months, 6-months and 1 year [16]. Due to lack of standardization in PFMT protocols and endpoints, individual studies may demonstrate significant results in a particular endpoint with no basis for comparison. In a non-randomized, retrospective study of 284 open radical prostatectomy patients, Patel analyzed time to continence in men undergoing physiotherapist-guided (PG) PFMT 4 weeks prior surgery versus the control group who received preoperative verbal instruction from the surgeon. At the 6-week time point, significantly fewer subjects in the PG-PFMT were incontinent as measured by a 24 h pad test [17]. A RCT by Centemero in 118 open radical prostatectomy patients, self-reported continence at 1 and 3-months was significantly different in patients who received PF-PFMT 4 weeks prior to surgery versus postoperative only. Additionally, the Quality of Life (QoL) from the International Continence Society male short form (ICSmalesf) was superior in the preoperative intervention group [12]. The available data suggests possible benefit in time to continence and patient satisfaction that are not fully analyzed in meta-analysis due to statistical limitations. However, the long-term benefit of preoperative PFMT has not been proven [18].

Pelvic Floor Stimulation: Electrical Stimulation [Transcutaneous Electrical Nerve Stimulation (TENS), Percutaneous Electrical Nerve Stimulation and Anal Stimulation] and Electromagnetic Therapy

Electrical stimulation (ES) of the pelvic floor is focused on stimulating motor fibers of the pelvic floor. It is unclear whether this solely acts by strengthening the periurethral musculature or whether it is also function as a form of biofeed-back [19–21]. Surface electrode placement may be transcutaneous or percutaneous [22–24]. Surface electrodes may be position in multiple locations: perianal, suprapubic, sacral dorsal penile and/or thigh. Percutaneous stimulation is primarily focused on posterior tibial nerve stimulation (PTENS). Stimulation protocols vary tremendously based on the following parameters: current source, pulse width and duration, current intensity (range), stimulus frequency, pulse shape, time and total number of sessions and rest to work ratio, type of urinary incontinence and type of electrical stimulation [22]. Direct rectal or anal stimulation has been used with the goal of directly simulating the pudendal nerve with elicitation of pelvic floor contraction. This modality is believed to be more efficacious in patients who demonstrated good pelvic floor control [25, 26]. Extracorporeal magnetic innervation (ExMI) was developed to allow for stimulation to the pelvic floor without the placement of surface electrodes or cavitary probes. The energy is delivered while in the sitting position through a padded seat containing the magnetic coils - Neocontrol (Neotonus, Inc., Marietta, GA).

Studies comparing groups of patients treated ES plus PFMT versus PFMT only tend to demonstrate benefit at 3- and 6-months but equivalence between groups at 1 year. Yamanishi randomized between postoperative anal surface electrode stimulation and PFMT versus written/verbal instruction PFMT only in 56 men post open radical prostatectomy. Combination therapy groups had significant improvement in 24 h pad test ICImale SF continence scores and Qol scores. However, these differences were not present at the 12 month time point [25]. Conversely, other series have reported an increased level of adverse events in patient receiving either rectal probe or perianal surface electrode ES [27]. Similar results are mirrored in ExMI literature; Koo randomized patients to ExMI or PMT starting 1 week after catheter removal. The ExMi group demonstrated decreased 24-h pad weight at 1 and 3 months post-op; this difference was no longer present at 6 months. Although the advantage in the ExMI group was not maintained, it does demonstrate a possible shortened time to continence [28].

Based on the failure to identify a clear sustained benefit for electrical stimulation over PMFT with the potential for increased adverse events, we currently do not uniformly utilize these forms of electrical stimulation in our continence rehabilitation program.

Lifestyle Adjustments

Behavioral modifications including diet, fluid management and weight loss have been demonstrated to be effective in significantly reducing daily urine loss [29]. Therefore, patients should be instructed to avoid caffeine and monitor their responses to acidic and spicy foods with the goal of eliminating bladder irritants. In addition to influencing leakage volume, weight has been linked to inferior outcomes of male incontinence procedures (slings and artificial urinary sphincter) [30, 31]. Optimization of comorbid conditions affecting urinary symptoms and incontinence is included in lifestyle modification. Improvement of diabetic management includes more rigid diet control and exercise. However, if the patient is unable to satisfactorily control his sugars with conservative measures collaboration with his endocrinologist or internist is required [32]. Total body conditioning has also gained attention as an adjunct to recovery of incontinence. Adjustment of diuretic timing can be critical to decreasing episodes of nocturnal enuresis. While all of these measures are intuitive and linked to reductions in urinary incontinence, there are no randomized studies testing lifestyle interventions to objective urinary outcomes.

Expectant Management/Watchful Waiting

Although data suggest that incontinence seems to stabilize at the 6-month point after robotic assisted radical prostatectomy, observational studies in the past have shown that a 10–15 % of patients may experience improvement up to 24 months [1, 33, 34]. Therefore, we are careful to ask whether the patient has experienced improvement within the last 4–6 weeks. In those with milder incontinence, continuation of pelvic floor muscle exercises combined with maximal lifestyle modification is a viable option. At any point, the management can be changed to a surgical intervention if the patient's progress stagnates or the level of bother exceeds his willingness to continue waiting.

Medical Management of Stress Incontinence

The primary management of male stress incontinence, especially severe incontinence, has not been pharmacological. However, there are categories of medications which have been studied for this purpose—alpha-adrenoceptor agonists, Beta 2-adrenoceptor agonists, and serotonin–noradrenaline reuptake inhibitors [35].

α-Adrenoceptor Agonists

Ephedrine, phenylpropanolamine and midodrine have been studied in distant past in mixed gender studies for use in stress urinary incontinence [36–38]. Though the studies were small, there were significant improvements in incontinence. Unfortunately, ephedrine is highly regulated and not approved for use in urinary incontinence. Phenylpropanolamine was pulled from the US market due to the risk of hemorrhagic stroke. Midodrine is available in the USA with approved indication of symptomatic orthostatic hypotension. However, there have been no recent studies evaluating its effectiveness for postprostatectomy incontinence. Anecdotally, the decongestant agents in Zyrtec D® and Seldane D®, pseudoephedrine, can be used on a prn basis for incontinence. However, this has not been evaluated in a clinical trial.

β₂-Adrenoceptor Agonists

Clenbuterolis a sympathomimetic amine used by sufferers of breathing disorders as a decongestant and bronchodilator. Although there are two studies evaluating its effectiveness for male stress urinary incontinence, there no randomized clinical trials in male patients [39, 40]. Currently, this agent is not approved for any indication by the FDA.

Serotonin–Noradrenaline Reuptake Inhibitors

The use of imipramine for urinary incontinence stems from initial usage in the pediatric population for nocturnal enuresis and combination agent for neurogenic detrusor overactivity. Studies in post-prostatectomy patients have been limited [41]. Duloxetine, a selective serotonin (5-HT) and norepinephrine (NE) reuptake inhibitor, decreases stress urinary incontinence by augmenting urethral sphincter contractility [42]. The drug inhibits the presynaptic reuptake of 5-HT and NE at Onuf's nucleus in the sacral spinal cord resulting in increased in rhabdosphincter activity due to increased postsynaptic receptor stimulation. In 2013, Neff reported on the usage of duloxetine in 94 post prostatectomy patients. While pad usage, IIQ-7 scores and QOL scores were statistically improved, 65 % of patients discontinued the medication due to side effects and/or lack of efficacy. While the agent is approved by the FDA for major depressive disorder, generalized anxiety disorder, fibromyalgia and neuropathic pain; it is not indicated for stress urinary incontinence.

Urethral Bulking Agents

Urethral bulking agents remain the least invasive surgical technique in the treatment of male stress urinary incontinence (SUI). The utilization of materials to improve urethral coaptation evolved from initial application in females for intrinsic sphincter deficiency (ISD) [43]. Development of the perfect injectable agent—durable, efficacious, easily injectable, and safe—is ongoing. Polytetrafluoroethylene (Teflon) was one of the first agents utilized; however, due to its particle size, migration occurred to regional lymph nodes, lungs, and brain. Consequently, Teflon was withdrawn from the market [44]. This clinical experience was utilized to guide the design of future synthetic injectable agents. Secondary to concerns associated with the migration of synthetic compounds, there was a natural interest in harvest and reinjection of an autologous substance. This reasoning formed the basis for the utilization of subcutaneous fat. Although it proved to be technically feasible in female patients, the success rates for the treatment of continence were poor [45].

Irrespective of gender, the most studied urethral bulking agent has been bovine collagen (Contigen®). Although no longer commercially available for urological applications in the USA, it served as the gold standard for efficacy. Currently, the most commonly used synthetic agents for urethral bulking are polydimethylsiloxane (Macroplastique®,Uroplasty, Minnetonka, MN, USA), carbon-coated zirconium oxide beads (Durasphere®,Carbon Medical Technologies Inc., St. Paul Minnesota) and hydroxylapatite spheres in carboxymethylcellulose carrier [Coaptite (Boston, MA, Boston Scientific Corporation)]. Secondarily, materials with primary indications for pediatric vesicoureteral reflux [Deflux (Q-Med, Uppsala, Sweden), Zuidex (Q-Med AB, Uppsala, Sweden)] have been studied for use for in female urethral bulking without demonstrating equivalence to bovine collagen [46]. While the success/improved rates range between 20 and 70 % in women, they are modest at best in male patients. Irrespective of gender, injectable therapy is a consideration in patients who are unable to tolerate or refuse more invasive surgical therapy. In male patients, the best success rates have been described in patients with a high Valsalva leak point pressure, unscarred vesicourethral anastomosis and no radia-

tion history (5, 6) [47, 48]. Each of these agents is discussed in further detail including methods of administration and available literature. No currently available agents have FDA approval for the treatment of male incontinence. However, Macroplastique® and Durasphere™ are approved outside of the USA for this indication.

Assessment

The minimum assessment prior to proceeding with injectable therapy consists of cystoscopic evaluation to confirm suitability of the anastomosis and proximal urethra. Scarred, noncompliant tissue will not accommodate the material resulting in a difficult and ineffective injection. Although urodynamic evaluation is routinely performed in the evaluation of post prostatectomy incontinence, its utility for predicting the success of anti-incontinence therapy has not been proven [49]. However, patients with complaints suggestive of detrusor overactivity and/or detrusor hypocontractility should be evaluated prior to proceeding.

Antimicrobial Prophylaxis

In the past, a 2–3 day course of oral antibiotics was recommended as appropriate course length for injectable therapy [50]. At a minimum, the AUA Best Practice Policy Statement for Antimicrobial Prophylaxis for Urological Procedures recommends a 24-h course of a fluoroquinolone or trimethoprim-sulfamethoxazole for cystoscopic procedures with manipulation [51].

General Technique

Antegrade and retrograde techniques have been utilized for the injection of bulking agents in the male patient. Periurethral and transurethral approaches are described as methods for delivery of injectable materials to the male bladder neck; however, the retrograde transurethral technique is accepted as the standard outpatient clinic approach. Therefore, we describe the use of bulking agents in this context.

Injection Basics

The posterior urethra is made up of four layers histologically; mucosa, lamina propria, muscularis, and adventitia. The lamina propria is the appropriate layer for urethral bulking agent injection as it contains the potential space where the product can be delivered [47]. In the postprostatectomy male this layer may be obliterated by scar just distal to the anastomosis secondary to prolonged catheterization, urine leak, or retropubic hematoma. All materials require a needle for delivery of the material into the submucosal space. The size of the needle is dependent on the characteristics of the agent. Materials composed of a larger average particle size and higher viscosity will require a larger gauge needle. In general, however, dedicated injection needles range in size from 18 to 22 gauge. A standard rigid cystoscope or an injection scope with a working element can be utilized (Table 3.3). Injection systems are currently available from the following cystoscopic equipment manufacturers: Richard Wolf (Fig. 3.7) and Karl Storz (Fig. 3.8). These systems allow for more precise guidance of the needle using a resectoscope element rather than making manual adjustments via the working channel.

Preparation for Injection

The patient is positioned in the dorsolithotomy position. The perineum is prepped and draped in a standard fashion. The urethra is infused with 20 cc of 2 % lidocaine jelly and allowed to dwell for at least 10 min after placement of a penile occlusive device. To improve analgesia, 1 % lidocaine solution (0.25–0.5 ml) may injected in the planned injection locations. Attempted re-cannulation of these needle sites for the bulking agent delivery decreases the likelihood of material extravasation from additional punctures in

the urethral mucosa. For all agents with the exception of Macroplastique®, it is possible to use the same needle for the local and injectable in series, thus reducing the possibility of creating multiple mucosal defects. Prior to placing the scope, the needle should be primed with local anesthetic and passed through the working channel.

Injection Technique

After navigating the penile and bulbar urethra, the bladder should be drained to decrease discomfort from over-distension during the procedure. Subsequently, the bladder neck is visualized and the scope is withdrawn 1.5–2.0 cm distally. Plan your injection sites after reassessing the quality of the bladder neck tissue. A standard location using a clock reference would be 4 and 8 o'clock in the male patient. Prior to mucosal penetration, confirm that the needle has been primed with local anesthetic. Alert the patient that he will feel a "stick followed a burning sensation then nothing." Using an analogy of oral local anesthetic for dental procedures may be helpful. Advance the needle through the urethral mucosa at a 45° angle to the lumen. The bevel of the needle should be directed towards the lumen. Due to limited potential volume in submucosal space, it is necessary to be judicious about the amount of local injected. Thus, limit the injected volume per site to 0.5 ml or less, if possible. After injection, request verbal feedback from the patient regarding when the discomfort has dissipated prior to proceeding. At this point, the local anesthetic syringe is switched for the injectable agent of choice (with the exception of Macroplastique). The unique technical variations for successful injection of each bulking agent are detailed below.

Post-procedure

The bladder should be sufficiently full from irrigation fluid for an immediate trial of voiding. In the event that the patient feels unable to empty completely or reports a weak stream, an ultrasound

Table 3.3 Injectable agents with equipment specifications

Injectable material	Trade name	Syringe sizes (ml)	Needle (manufacturer, product #)
Polydimethylsiloxane	Macroplastique	2.5	Rigid endoscopic needle-3.8 Fr. shaft × 14.5″ (370 mm) long with 20 gauge tip × 0.54″ (14 mm) long (Uroplasty: MRN420) Uroplasty rigid endoscopic needle 5 Fr. shaft × 15″ (380 mm) long with 18 gauge tip × 0.54″ (14 mm) long (Uroplasty: MRN520)
Carbon coated zirconium oxide	Durasphere	1 and 3	Bent spinal tip, 15 in., 18 gauge (Coloplast: 890205) Needle: pencil point tip, 15 in., 20 gauge (Coloplast: 890209)
Calcium hydroxylapatite (CaHA) and sodium carboxymethylcellulose (NaCMC)	Coaptite	1	Sidekick™ needle 14.6 in., 21 gauge (Boston Scientific: M0068903040)
Glutaraldehyde cross-linked bovine collagen	Contigen	2.5	Rigid endoscopic needle—22 gauge (Richard Wolfe)

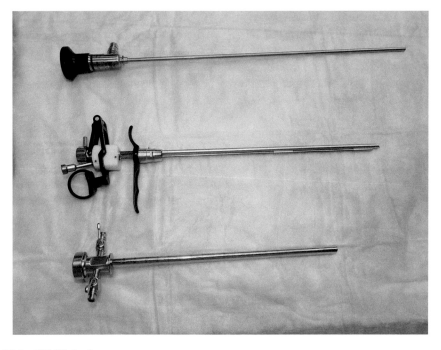

Fig. 3.7 Richard Wolf injection scope

bladder volume index is performed. Urinary retention may be treated with either intermittent catheterization or a small Foley catheter. Due to concerns of displacing or distorting the achieved coaptation with the Foley catheter, the preferred option would be intermittent catheterization.

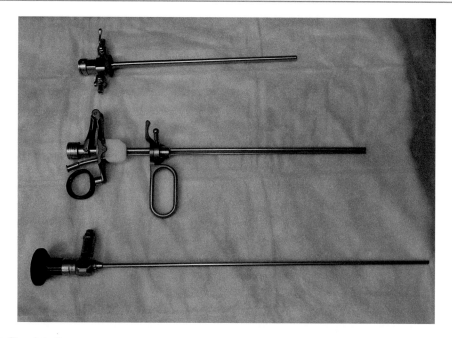

Fig. 3.8 Storz injection scope

Re-injection

Determination of the results from the injection are made after any local anesthetic has dissipated along with any accompanying swelling—7–10 days. Further injections are deferred until about 6–8 weeks by which point the injections sites are sufficiently healed.

Injectable Agents

Biologics

Bovine Collagen

Although bovine collagen is not currently available for urological applications in the USA, it served as the comparator for the majority of currently available agents. Thus a brief discussion of its prior usage is an important foundation for newer agents.

Contigen® (C. R. Bard, Covington, GA) glutaraldehyde cross-linked (GAX) collagen received US Food and Drug Administration (FDA) approval in 1993 for the treatment of Intrinsic Sphincter Deficiency (ISD); however, distribution was discontinued in 2011 by the manufacturer. Contigen® was composed primarily from bovine, Type I collagen which is typically found in bone, cartilage and connective tissue of cattle. The extracted collagen was then purified and cross-linked with glutaraldehyde (GAX) mixed in a phosphate buffered saline to make up the injectable compound. After injection GAX collagen starts degrading within 12 weeks and ultimately completely degrades within 9–19 months. Although the injected collagen has been demonstrated to promote intraurethral collagen production, however, several studies have shown the need for reinjection to maintain continence, thereby necessitating booster injections.

As a bovine byproduct, allergic reactions were a major concern and interestingly were predominately found in females [52]. McClelland et al. 1996 reported that 28 % of patients who had intraurethral collagen injections for urinary incontinence produced specific antibodies against bovine dermal collagen [53]. Furthermore, Dmochowski et al. 2000 reported allergic reactions in approximately 4 % of females [54]. Although 70 % of positive reactions are identified within 3 days, 30 % may not be expressed until 4 weeks [55]. Delayed allergic reactions associated with arthralgias were also reported by Stothers et al. 1998 [55]. Therefore, pre-injection skin testing is an absolute requirement with an interval of one full month prior to injection to allow for detection of delayed reactions.

Collagen Efficacy

Under the best circumstances, less than 20 % of postprostatectomy males achieve a dry state with collagen [56, 57]. In the largest published study of the utilization of collage for male stress urinary incontinence, the outcomes of 322 patients were analyzed. Overall improvement was reported in approximately 50 % with a mean duration of 6 months whereas complete continence was achieved in 17 % with a mean duration of 8.87 months. Of note 1.5 % of patients reported an increase in incontinence following collagen injections [58].

Synthetic Injectables

Durasphere®

Product Description

Durasphere® is a non-immunogenic, nonpyrogenic, nonabsorbable urethral bulking agent made of pyrolytic carbon coated zirconium oxide beads with suspended in a water-gel with 2.8 % beta-glucan (Fig. 3.9). Inert and non-immunogenic, a skin test is not necessary prior to the procedure. The initial formulation of the agent was hampered by large particle sizes with the beads ranging from 212 to 500 μm requiring a larger gauge needle to facilitate injection. Technical problems triggered further evolution leading to the production of Durasphere® EXP (Coloplast, Inc., Minneapolis, MN). The current agent is primarily differentiated by graphite coating and smaller beads (90–212 μm) allowing for injection with a 20 gauge needle. Thus, treatment in the outpatient clinic setting is much more feasible.

Durasphere® EXP is available in 3 ml syringes for periurethral injections (for women) and 1 ml syringes for transurethral injections. Additionally,

the manufacturer distributes 15 in. 18 gauge (bent spinal tip) and 20 gauge (pencil point tip) needles for transurethral injections (Fig. 3.10).

Specific Tips and Manufacturer's Recommendations for Injection of Durasphere

After injection of the local anesthetic and connection of the Durasphere to the needle, the options are to: (1) retract the needle from the urethral mucosa, prime with the Durasphere followed by replacement of the needle in the same location or (2) keep the needle in-situ while injecting the anesthetic in the needle followed by the Durasphere. In the interest of minimizing manipulation and potential expansion of the puncture site, the latter is preferable.

In the post-prostatectomy patient, the length of supramembranous urethra is highly variable. Despite this, injection site must be selected with an entry point 1–1.5 cm distal to the bladder neck. The needle is oriented as previously described and advanced in the submucosal layer until the black hatch mark on the needle (1 cm from the bevel). Injection should be initiated with light pressure on the syringe plunger.

Injection of Durasphere can be technically challenging in the male patient due to the composition of the material. The potential space for injection must be compliant, expanding easily with little pressure on the syringe. If scarring is present requiring increased force to be applied to the syringe plunger, the beads and carrier solution will travel not through the needle at equivalent rates, resulting in the carrier solution advancing ahead of the beads. In the absence of the gel, the beads are unable to progress through the needle resulting in obstruction of the needle and syringe with the remaining beads. However, in patients with a compliant supramembranous urethra, 2–3 ml of Durasphere is required for injection.

If anything more than light consistent pressure is necessary, the best course of action is reorientation of the needle to identify an optimal space. The first option is retraction of the needle by 0.5 cm followed by redirection into a slightly deeper plane. In the event this maneuver is not

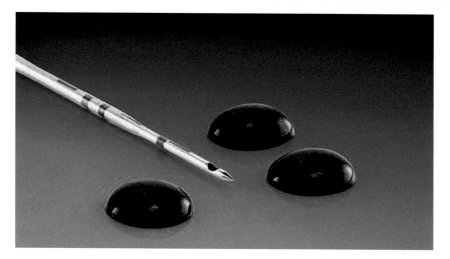

Fig. 3.9 Durasphere material

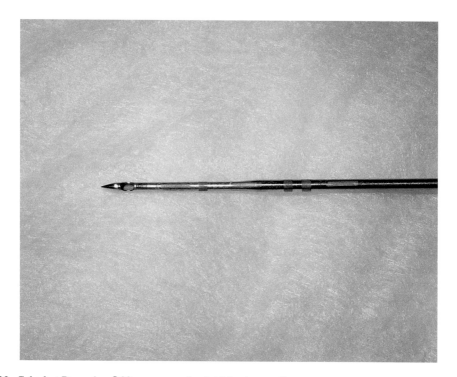

Fig. 3.10 Coloplast Durasphere® 20 gauge, pencil point injection needle

successful, the needle should be withdrawn completely. Prior to identifying an alternate location, advance the scope in the bladder to assure easy flow of the agent in the absence of resistance. If the needle has become obstructed, remove the needle to allow examination on the back table. A replacement needle will be necessary if the lumen is not cleared successfully.

Once a suitable location for injection is secured, injection usually proceeds in 1–2 additional locations using 1 ml per site. After completing injection at each location, the needle is left stationary for 10–15 s prior to withdrawing the needle. Once overall satisfactory coaptation is achieved, the scope is removed. Rather than passing the scope into the bladder for drainage, the bladder is left to full to allow for an immediate voiding trial as discussed previously.

Available Literature

Although the literature about Durasphere injections in women is ample, it is virtually nonexistent in males likely due to the increased technical difficulty and low success rates. Secin et al. discussed the efficacy of Durasphere in the treatment of mild to moderate post prostatectomy urinary incontinence in eight patients. The mean age of the patients was 63.2 years and median time of injection after radical prostatectomy was 25 months. The mean Durasphere volume injected was 23.8 ml with a median follow-up of 5 months. Only three patients reported subjective transient improvement and five patients opted for more invasive surgical option. One patient reported worsening of his incontinence and another had acute urinary retention requiring an indwelling catheter for 4 days [59].

Coaptite®

Product Description

Coaptite® is a non-pyrogenic, non-immunogenic agent composed of calcium hydroxylapatite (CaHA) spheres suspended in an aqueous based gel carrier of sodium carboxymethylcellulose (NaCMC) and glycerin. Since CaHA is a naturally occurring substance in the human body, pre-procedural skin testing is not required. Similar to Durasphere, Coaptite is radiopaque allowing visualization on imaging. With mean bead diameter of 100 µm (range, 75–125 µm), the particles are large enough to minimize migration risks but small enough to allow for smooth injection using a 21 gauge needle. The material is supplied in 1 ml syringes with no additional equipment needed other than a standard cystoscope for the injection procedure. Common side-effects include hematuria, dysuria, UTI, urgency, uri-

nary retention with few cases of erosion and urethral prolapse reported in female patients. To date, there is no literature available for the treatment of urinary incontinence in males.

Specific Tips and Manufacturer's Recommendations for Injection of Coaptite

Coaptite has some similarity to Durasphere due the particle and carrier/gel composition of the material. However, due to the particle size, Coaptite is suitable for a injection with a slightly smaller needle. Although there is less risk of separation between the calcium hydroxyapatite spheres and the carrier, the same caution should be taken as described with Durasphere (Fig. 3.11a–c).

Macroplastique®

Product Description

Macroplastique®, a newer urethral bulking agent, is composed of vulcanized polydimethylsiloxane (a solid silicone elastomer) suspended in a bio-excretable polyvinylpyrrolidone (PVP) carrier gel pre-packaged in sterile 2.5 ml syringes. Polydimethylsiloxane (PDS) is a large molecule with a mean diameter of 140 µm that upon implantation becomes encapsulated in fibrin and collagen therefore minimizing the risk of migration. However, due to its size and associated viscosity, special equipment is required for particle delivery [60, 61].

Specific Tips and Manufacturer's Recommendations for Injection of Macroplastique®

Injection of Macroplastique® requires a reusable Administration Device which includes a syringe adapter (Fig. 3.12). The physician can choose one of two needles to attach to the adapter for product delivery; (1) Uroplasty Rigid Endoscopic Needle 3.8 Fr. shaft × 14.5″ (370 mm) long with 20 gauge tip × 0.54″ (14 mm) long or (2) Uroplasty Rigid Endoscopic Needle 5 Fr. shaft × 15″ (380 mm) long with 18 gauge

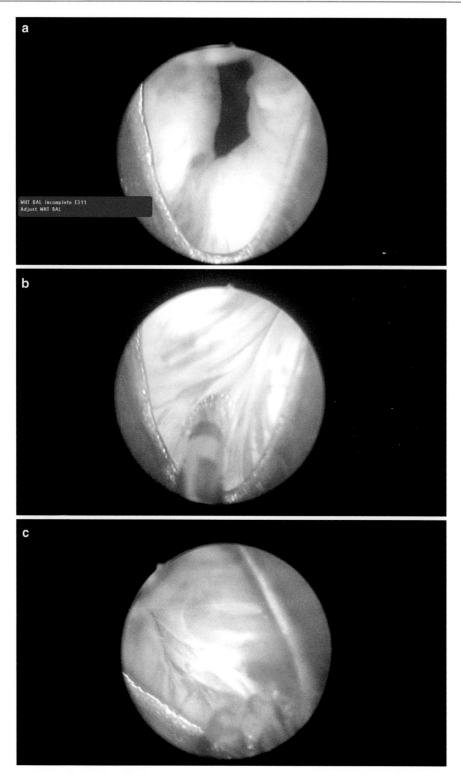

Fig. 3.11 (**a**) Open bladder neck pre-Coaptite Injection; (**b**) Transurethral injection needle placement; (**c**) Coapted bladder neck post-injection

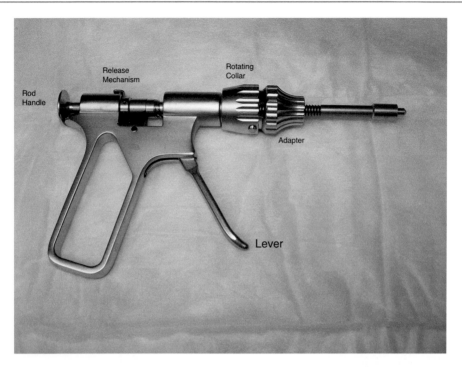

Fig. 3.12 Macroplastique administration device

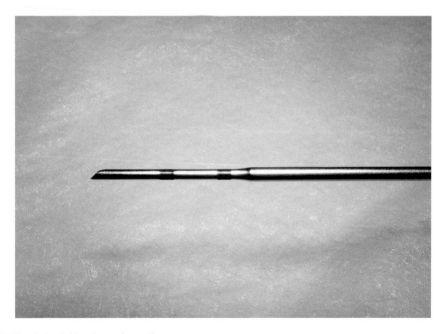

Fig. 3.13 Uroplasty rigid endoscopic needle

tip×0.54″ (14 mm) long (Fig. 3.13). Recent modifications in the dimensions and weight of the Administration device make it possible for a single person to manage the scope and the device in comparison with earlier models [62].

Preparation of the Macroplastique Administration Device

The Macroplastique syringe plunger is placed into the syringe collar. The syringe collar assembly is locked by rotating the hub of the

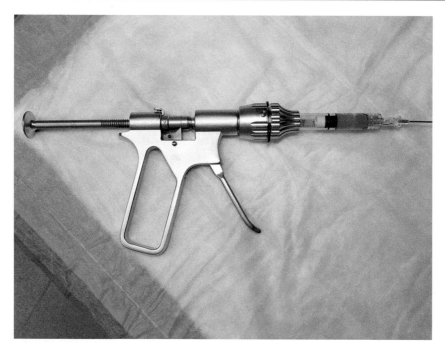

Fig. 3.14 Macroplastique device loaded with syringe and needle

Administration Device. The selected Uroplasty needle is attached to the luer lock of the syringe and rotated to achieve a tight connection. The protective sleeve from the needle is removed. Prime the needle with Macroplastique by engaging the Administration Device. To stop the flow, depress the release mechanism located on top of the Administration Device (Fig. 3.14).

Injection

Prior to bulking, adequate analgesia must be established. The most efficient manner to achieve this consists of injecting the local anesthetic in all planned injection sites prior to starting with the Macroplastique. As previously mentioned, it is necessary to attempt to reutilize the same sites for the bulking agent to prevent additional areas for extravasation.

During placement of the needle and Administration Device through the working channel, it may be necessary for an assistant to stabilize the cystoscope. Advance the scope into the bladder while pushing the needle forward to con-firm orientation of the bevel towards the lumen. Retract the needle tip and scope back into the ure-thra 1.5 to 2.0 cm distal from the bladder neck. For injection, the manufacturer describes a "tissue tunneling" technique which is similar to the ideal placement technique for all injectables. The nee-dle enters the tissue at a 30–45° angle followed by advancement of the needle for 0.5 cm. The angle is the flattened to be parallel with the urethra and the needle is advanced for another 0.5 cm.

The Administration Device lever should be deployed slowly to prevent rapid egress of the agent into the submucosa. Pause a few seconds between each pull to allow for equilibration of the pressure within the submucosal space. Continue until the syringe is completed at each location and/or satisfactory coaptation has been achieved. In all positions, wait approximately 30 s before withdrawing the needle from the tissue to limit product loss from the implantation site. It is suggested that further injections not be attempted until after 12 weeks from the prior injection.

Published Data

Macroplastique® has been studied extensively in females; however, there are few studies in males which deserve mention. Kylmala et al. studied 50 patients with mild to moderate post prostatectomy SUI. Macroplastique was injected at 5 o'clock or 7 o'clock or both with repeated injections being at least 3 months apart. After the first treatment, 6 patients were completely dry and 28 reported improvement after which 40 patients had a second treatment and an additional 10 patients became dry. Third and fourth injections were given to 23 and 8 patients out of whom 9 and 5 patients became dry, respectively. The total mean volume of Macroplastique used was 7.1 ml, with a mean of three injections with a mean follow-up of 7.3 months. The overall dry rate was 60 % and improvement in 28 % with adverse effects that included dysuria with no reported Acute Urinary Retention (AUR) [63].

Imamoglu et al. divided 45 patients with PPI into two groups by severity of incontinence, group I (21 patients) had minimal incontinence and group II (24 patients) had total incontinence. The patients in each group were then randomized to get AUS (11 and 11) vs. Macroplastique injection (10 and 13). The mean follow-up for AUS patients was 60 months vs. 48 months for the Macroplastique patients. The dry rate in group I was 90 % in AUS patients and 80 % in injection patients with no statistically significant difference. However, group II demonstrated a significant difference ($p<0.01$) with a dry rate of 72.7 % vs. 23.1 % for AUS and injection patients, respectively. Injections were performed at 3, 6, and 9 o'clock with a mean number of injections of 1.2 and a mean injection volume of 11.9 ml (5–7.5 ml each injection); a 4.3 % AUR rate was reported [64]. Lee et al. 2014 studied 30 patients with PPI and evaluated Macroplastique® single injection treatment with a mean follow-up of 9.3 months. Injections were performed at 3, 6, 9, and 12 o'clock with a mean injection volume of 5.3 ml. The success rate was reported as 43.3 % with a complete dry rate of 10 % and AUR rate of 16.7 %. Though not significant, the success rate was higher in non-radiated patients with a lower LPP [60].

The most common adverse effects of Macroplastique include urinary retention (5.9–17.5 %), urinary frequency (0–72.4 %), dysuria (0–100 %), and rarely UTI (0–6.25 %).

Agents Used Primarily Used for Other Urologic Applications

The same injectable agents employed as a treatment for vesicoureteral reflux in the pediatric population have been used with variable success for PPI.

Deflux®

Product Description

Deflux® is a sterile, mixture of viscous dextranomer microspheres (50 mg/ml) in a carrier gel of stabilized hyaluronic acid (15 mg/ml). The hyaluronic acid along with additional hydrogel/polysaccharide serves to improve delivery of the dextranomer microspheres. As hyaluronic acid has remarkable viscoelastic properties, it allows the mixture to be injected utilizing a needle as small as 23 gauge. The dextranomer microspheres have a mean diameter of 130 μm ranging between 80 and 250 μm. After injection, the hyaluronic acid is dissolved in the tissue within 2 weeks leaving the dextranomer microspheres in place as the main bulking agent. It was originally designed for SUI in women, however, bovine collagen had more favorable outcomes. Due to its unparalleled safety profile, its use in children continues for both incontinence and vesicoureteral reflux [65].

Deflux® is manufactured in 1 ml glass syringes equipped with luer lock fitting, a tip cap, plunger and plunger rod. It can be injected using a standard cystoscope with a 23 gauge needle. It is injected submucosally in the standard fashion until complete coaptation is noted.

Zuidex™ implacement therapy also a hyaluronic acid/dextranomer copolymer designed for SUI in the USA was discontinued after a large multicenter study was showed increased incidence of sterile abscess formation.

Mode of Delivery and Manufacturer Instructions

As per the manufacturer, it is recommended to use the Deflux metal needle (3.7 F × 23G tip × 350 mm) for safe and accurate administration of Deflux. However, any needle with 23 or 22 gauge could be safely utilized.

Similarly to Coaptite and Collagen, only a standard cystoscope is needed with an injection element. Deflux can then be injected at the bladder neck or pre-sphincteric urethra submucosally at three sites until coaptation is seen. Injecting 6 ml or more is not recommended as no studies demonstrated safety at higher volumes.

Published Data

Deflux® is not typically used as first line urethral bulking agent in adults however, several studies have been conducted in children particularly those who wish to avoid major reconstructive surgery. Lottmann et al. studied 61 children (41 males and 20 females) most of which were in diapers due to severe sphincteric incompetence, exstrophy-epispadias, neuropathic bladder, and ectopic ureters. The mean age was 10.3 years and the mean injection volume of Deflux was 3.9 cc (range 1.6–12) with a follow-up after the last injection was 6–84 months (mean 28). The group noted at 1 month 79 % of the patients were dry or improved. At 6 months 56 % were dry or improved. Longer term follow-up at 1 year, 3 years, 4 years, and 7 years yielded a dry or improved rate of 52 %, 52 %, 48 %, and 40 % respectively [66].

Caione et al. in 2002 studied 16 patients with mean age of 10.6 years with a mean injection volume of 2.8 ml and a mean number of injections of 2.3. The mean pretreatment dry time was 35 min; however, it was 78, 80, and 74 min at 6 months, 12 months, and 24 months, respectively [67].

Misseri et al. 2005 studied a total of 16 patients (6 males and 10 females) ranging in age from 4 to 18 years with a mean follow-up of 9.5 months (range 3–24 months). The mean injected volume was 1.88 ml (range 0.8–4.4 ml) where complete dryness was noted in three patients, five patients were improved (all of which had catheterizable

channels) and eight patients showed no improvement at follow-up [68].

References

1. Sanda MG, Dunn RL, Michalski J, Sandler HM, Northouse L, Hembroff L, Lin X, Greenfield TK, Litwin MS, Saigal CS, Mahadevan A, Klein E, Kibel A, Pisters LL, Kuban D, Kaplan I, Wood D, Ciezki J, Shah N, Wei JT. Quality of life and satisfaction with outcome among prostate-cancer survivors. N Engl J Med. 2008;358(12):1250–61.
2. Newman DK, Guzzo T, Lee D, Jayadevappa R. An evidence-based strategy for the conservative management of the male patient with incontinence. Curr Opin Urol. 2014;24(6):553–9.
3. Wilson L, Brown JS, Shin GP, Luc KO, Subak LL. Annual direct cost of urinary incontinence. Obstet Gynecol. 2001;98:398–406.
4. Yamasato K, Kaneshiro B, Oyama IA. A simulation comparing thecost-effectiveness of adult incontinence products. J Wound Ostomy Continence Nurs. 2014;41(5):467–72.
5. Cooperberg MR, Master VA, Carroll PR. Health related quality of life significance of single pad urinary incontinence following radical prostatectomy. J Urol. 2003;170(2 Pt 1):512–5.
6. Moore KN, Schieman S, Ackerman T, Dzus HY, Metcalfe JB, Voaklander DC. Assessing comfort, safety, and patient satisfaction with three commonly used penile compression devices. Urology. 2004;63(1):150–4.
7. Kyle G. The use of urinary sheaths in male incontinence. Br J Nurs. 2011;20(6):338.
8. Robinson J. Continence: sizing and fitting a penile sheath. Br J Community Nurs. 2006;1(10):420–7.
9. Foratos DL, Sonke GS, Rapidou CA, Alivizatos GJ, Deliveliotis C, Constantinides CA, et al. Biofeedback versus verbal feedback as learning tools for pelvic muscle exercises in the early management of urinary incontinence after radical prostatectomy. BJU Int. 2002;89(7):714–9.
10. Moore KN, Valiquette L, Chetner MP, Byrniak S, Herbison GP. Return to continence after radical retropubic prostatectomy: a randomized trial of verbal and written instructions versus therapist-directed pelvic floor muscle therapy. Urology. 2008;72(6):1280–6.
11. Glazener C, Boachie C, Buckley B, Cochran C, Dorey G, Grant A, et al. Urinary incontinence in men after formal one-to-one pelvic-floor muscle training following radical prostatectomy or transurethral resection of the prostate (MAPS): two parallel randomized controlled trials. Lancet. 2011;378(9788):328–37.
12. Bales GT, Gerber GS, Minor TX, Mhoon DA, McFarland JM, Kim HL, Brendler CB. Effect of preoperative biofeedback/pelvic floor training on conti-

nence in men undergoing radical prostatectomy. Urology. 2000;56:627–30.

13. Centemero A, Rigatti L, Giraudo D, Lazzeri M, Lughezzani G, Zugna D, Montorsi F, Rigatti P, Guazzoni G. Preoperative pelvic floor muscle exercise for early continence after radical prostatectomy: a randomized controlled study. Eur Urol. 2010;57:1039–43.

14. Geraerts I, Van Poppel H, Devoogdt N, Joniau S, Van Cleynenbreugel B, De Groef A, Van Kampen M. Influence of preoperative and postoperative pelvic floor muscle training (PFMT) compared with postoperative PFMT on urinary incontinence after radical prostatectomy: a randomized controlled trial. Eur Urol. 2013;64:766–72.

15. Dijkstra-Eshuis J, Van den Bos TW, Splinter R, Bevers RF, Zonneveld WC, Putter H, Pelger RC, Voorham-van der Zalm PJ. Effect of preoperative pelvic floor muscle therapy with biofeedback versus standard care on stress urinary incontinence and quality of life in men undergoing laparoscopic radical prostatectomy: a randomised control trial. Neurourol Urodyn. 2015;34(2):144–50.

16. Wang W, Huang QM, Liu FP, Mao QQ. Effectiveness of preoperative pelvic floor muscle training for urinary incontinence after radical prostatectomy: a meta-analysis. BMC Urol. 2014;14:99.

17. Patel MI, Yao J, Hirschhorn AD, Mungovan SF. Preoperative pelvic floor physiotherapy improves continence after radical retropubic prostatectomy. Int J Urol. 2013;20:986–92.

18. Anderson CA, Omar MI, Campbell SE, Hunter KF, Cody JD, Glazener CM. Conservative management for postprostatectomy urinary incontinence. Cochrane Database Syst Rev. 2015;1, CD001843.

19. Fall M, Lindstrom S. Functional electrical stimulation: physiological basis and clinical principles. Int Urogynecol J Pelvic Floor Dysfunct. 1994;5:296–304.

20. Hay-Smith J, Berghmans B, Burgio K, Dumoulin C, Hagen S, Moore K, et al. Adult conservative management. In: Abrams P, Cardozo L, Khoury S, Wein A, editors. Incontinence: 4th international consultation on incontinence. Recommendations of the International Scientific Committee: evaluation and treatment of urinary incontinence, pelvic organ prolapse and faecal incontinence: Paris, France, July 5-9, 2008. Plymouth, UK: Health Publication Ltd; 2009. p. 1025–120.

21. Berghmans LCM, Bernards ATM, Bluyssen AMW, Grupping-Morel MHM, Hendriks HJM, de Jong-van Ierland MJEA, et al. Dutch physiotherapy guidelines for stress urinary incontinence [KNGF–richtlijn Stress urine–incontinentie]. Nederland Tijdschrift voor Fysiotherapie. 1998;108 Suppl 4:1–35.

22. Berghmans LCM, Van Waalwijk van Doorn ESC, Nieman FHM, De Bie RA, Van den Brandt PA, Van Kerrebroeck PEV. Efficacy of physical therapeutic modalities in womenwith proven bladder overactivity. Eur Urol. 2002;41:581–8.

23. Govier FE, Litwiller S, Nitti V, Kreder Jr KJ, Rosenblatt P. Percutaneous afferent neuromodulation for the refractoryoveractive bladder: results of a multicenter study. J Urol. 2001;165(4):1193–8.

24. van Balken MR, Vandoninck V, Gisolf KWH, Vergunst H, Kiemeney LALM, Debruyne FMJ, et al. Posterior tibial nerve stimulation as neuro modulative treatment of lower urinary tract dysfunction. J Urol. 2001;166(3):914–8.

25. Yamanishi T, Mizuno T, Watanabe M, Honda M, Yoshida K. Randomized, placebo controlled study of electrical stimulation with pelvic floor muscle training for severe urinary incontinence after radical prostatectomy. J Urol. 2010;184:2007–12.

26. Yokoyama T, Nishiguchi J, Watanabe T, Nose H, Nozaki K, Fujita O, et al. Comparative study of effects of extracorporeal magnetic innervation versus electrical stimulation for urinary incontinence after radical prostatectomy. Urology. 2004;63(2):264–7.

27. Hoffman W, Liedke S, Dombo O, Otto U. Electrical stimulation for post-operative stress urinary incontinence [Die Elektrostimulation in der Therapie der Postoperativen Harninkontinenz]. Urologe. 2005;1:33–40.

28. Koo D, So SM, Lim JS. Effect of extracorporeal magnetic innervation (ExMI) pelvic floor therapy on urinary incontinence after radical prostatectomy. Korean J Urol. 2009;50(1):23–7.

29. Maserejian NN, Wager CG, Giovannucci EL, et al. Intake of caffeinated, carbonated, or citrus beverage types and development of lower urinary tract symptoms in men and women. Am J Epidemiol. 2013;177:1399–410.

30. Wang R, McGuire EJ, He C, Faerber GJ, Latini JM. Long-term outcomes after primary failures of artificial urinary sphincter implantation. Urology. 2012;79(4):922–8.

31. Leruth J, Waltregny D, de Leval J. The inside-out transobturator male sling for the surgical treatment of stress urinary incontinence after radical prostatectomy: midterm results of a single-center prospective study. Eur Urol. 2012;61(3):608–15.

32. Breyer BN, Phelan S, Hogan PE, et al. Look AHEAD Research Group. Intensive lifestyle intervention reduces urinary incontinence in overweight/obese men with type 2 diabetes: results from the Look AHEAD Trial. J Urol. 2014;192:144–9.

33. Lepor H, Kaci L, Xue X. Continence following radical retropubic prostatectomy using self-reporting instruments. J Urol. 2004;171(3):1212–5.

34. Ficarra V, Novara G, Rosen RC, et al. Systematic review and meta-analysis of studies reporting urinary continence recovery after robot-assisted radical prostatectomy. Eur Urol. 2012;62:405–17.

35. Tsakiris P, de la Rosette JJ, Michel MC, Oelke M. Pharmacologic treatment of male stress urinary

incontinence: systematic review of the literature and levels of evidence. Eur Urol. 2008;53:53–9.

36. Diokno AC, Taub M. Ephedrine in treatment of urinary incontinence. Urology. 1975;5:624–5.

37. Awad SA, Downie JW, Kiruluta HG. Alpha-adrenergic agents in urinary disorders of the proximal urethra. Part I Sphincteric incontinence. Br J Urol. 1978;50:332–5.

38. Nito H. Clinical effect of midodrine hydrochloride on the patients with urinary incontinence. Hinyokika Kiyo. 1994;40:91–4.

39. Noguchi M, Eguchi Y, Ichiki J, Yahara J, Noda S. Therapeutic efficacy of clenbuterol for urinary incontinence after radical prostatectomy. Int J Urol. 1997;4:480–3.

40. Zozikov B, Kunchev SI, Varlev C. Application of clenbuterol in the treatment of urinary incontinence. Int Urol Nephrol. 2001;33:413–6.

41. Reid GF, Fitzpatrick JM, Worth PH. The treatment of patients with urinary incontinence after prostatectomy. Br J Urol. 1980;52:532–4.

42. Schlenker B, Gratzke C, Reich O, et al. Preliminary results on the off-label use of duloxetine for the treatment of stress incontinence after radical prostatectomy or cystectomy. Eur Urol. 2006;49:1075–8.

43. Elsergany R, Elgamasy AN, Ghoniem GM. Transurethral collagen injection for female stress incontinence. Int Urogynecol J Pelvic Floor Dysfunct. 1998;9(1):13–8.

44. Herschorn S, Glazer AA. Early experience with small volume periurethral polytetrafluoroethylene for female stress urinary incontinence. J Urol. 2000;163(6):1838–42.

45. Cervigni M, Tomiselli G, Perricone C, et al. Endoscopic treatment of sphincter insufficiency with autologous fat injection. Arch Ital Urol Androl. 1994;66:219–24.

46. Lightner D, Rovner E, Corcos J, et al. Randomized controlled multisite trial of injected bulking agents for women with intrinsic sphincter deficiency: mid-urethral injection of Zuidex via the Implacer versus proximal urethral injection of Contigen cystoscopically. Urology. 2009;74:771–5.

47. Cespedes RD, Leng WW, McGuire EJ. Collagen injection therapy for postprostatectomy incontinence. Urology. 1999;54:597.

48. Kim PH, Pinheiro LC, Atoria CL, Eastham JA, Sandhu JS, Elkin EB. Trends in the use of incontinence procedures after radical prostatectomy: a population based analysis. J Urol. 2013;189(2): 602–8.

49. Hosker G, Rosier P, Gajewski J, et al. Dynamic testing. In: Abrams P, Cardozo L, Khoury S, Wein A, editors. Incontinence—4th international consultation. Paris: Health Publications; 2009. p. 413–522.

50. Appell RA, Winters JC. Injection therapy for urinary incontinence. In: Wein A, Kavoussi LR, Novick AC, editors. Campbell-Walsh urology. Philadelphia: Saunders Elsevier; 2007. p. 2272–87.

51. Wolf JS, Bennett CJ, Dmochowski R, et al. Best practice policy statement on urologic surgery antimicrobial prophylaxis. J Urol. 2008;179:1379–90.

52. Lightner DJ, Fox J, Klingele C. Cystoscopic injections of dextranomer hyaluronic acid into proximal urethra for urethral incompetence: efficacy and adverse outcomes. Urology. 2010;75(6):1310–4.

53. McClelland M, DeLustro F. Evaluation of antibody class in response to bovine collagen treatment in patients with urinary incontinence. J Urol. 1996;155:2068.

54. Dmochowski RR, Appell RA. Injectable agents in the treatment of stress urinary incontinence in women: where are we now? Urology. 2000;56(6 Suppl 1):32–40.

55. Keefe J, Wauk L, Chu S, et al. Clinical use of injectable bovine collagen: a decade of experience. Clin Mater. 1992;9:155–62.

56. Stothers L, Goldenberg SL. Delayed hypersensitivity and systemic arthralgia following transurethral collagen injection for stress urinary incontinence. J Urol. 1998;159(5):1507–9.

57. Faerber GJ, Richardson TD. Long-term results of transurethral collagen injection in men with intrinsic sphincter deficiency. J Endourol. 1997;11(4):273–7.

58. Westney OL, Bevan-Thomas R, Palmer JL, Cespedes RD, McGuire EJ. Transurethral collagen injections for male intrinsic sphincter deficiency: the University of Texas-Houston experience. J Urol. 2005;174(3):994–7.

59. Secin FP, Martínez-Salamanca JI, Eilber KS. Limited efficacy of permanent injectable agents in the treatment of stress urinary incontinence after radical prostatectomy. Arch Esp Urol. 2005;58(5):431–6.

60. Lee SW, Kang JH, Sung HH, Jeong US, Lee YS, Baek M, Lee KS. Treatment outcomes of transurethral macroplastique injection for postprostatectomy incontinence. Korean J Urol. 2014;55(3):182–9.

61. Ghoniem G, Corcos J, Comiter C, Westney OL, Herschorn S. Durability of bulking agent injection for female stress urinary incontinence: 2-year multicenter study results. J Urol. 2010;183(4):1444–9.

62. Uroplasty Macroplastique® Instructions Use. https://www.uroplasty.com/healthcarc/macroplastique

63. Kylmälä T, Tainio H, Raitanen M, Tammela TL. Treatment of postoperative male urinary incontinence using transurethral macroplastique injections. J Endourol. 2003;17:113–5.

64. Imamoglu MA, Tuygun C, Bakirtas H, Yigitbasi O, Kiper A. The comparison of artificial urinary sphyncter implantation and endourethral macroplastique injection for the treatment of postprostatectomy incontinence. Eur Urol. 2005;47:209–13.

65. Henly DR, Barrett DM, Weiland TL, O'Connor MK, Malizia AA, Wein AJ. Particulate silicone for use in periurethral injections: local tissue effects and search for migration. J Urol. 1995;153:2039–43.

66. Lottmann HB, Margaryan M, Lortat-Jacob S, Bernuy M, Läckgren G. Long-term effects of

dextranomer endoscopic injections for the treatment of urinary incontinence: an update of a prospective study of 61 patients. J Urol. 2006;176(4 Pt 2):1762–6.

67. Caione P, Capozza N. Endoscopic treatment of urinary incontinence in pediatric patients: 2-year experience with dextranomer/hyaluronic acid copolymer. J Urol. 2002;168(4 Pt 2):1868–71.

68. Misseri R, Casale AJ, Cain MP, Rink RC. Alternative uses of dextranomer/hyaluronic acid copolymer: the efficacy of bladder neck injection for urinary incontinence. J Urol. 2005;174(4 Pt 2):1691–3. discussion 1693-4.

Urinary Dysfunction in Prostate Cancer: Male Slings

4

Ricarda M. Bauer

For decades, the artificial urinary sphincter (AUS) was the gold standard for surgical treatment of persistent post-prostatectomy stress urinary incontinence (PPI). In the early 1960s, the first male slings were described by Berry and Kaufman and later by Schaeffer [1–3]. However, these slings were not widely used—mainly due to lack of published data, low success rates and high complications rates. Beginning in the late 1990s, new male slings were introduced.

Current available male slings systems can be classified into two subtypes: fixed slings and adjustable sling systems.

In recent years male slings have gained much popularity due to good functional results and low complications. In addition, patients' demand on minimally invasive treatment options restoring the natural voiding pattern is high and the opportunity to avoid using a mechanical device as the artificial sphincter is preferable to undergoing a for decades established treatment [4].

According to the current guidelines, male slings are an alternative for men with persistent stress urinary incontinence (grade of recommendation: C; level of evidence: 3) [5, 6].

With an increasing number of options available for the surgical treatment of PPI, it is important to be aware of available therapeutic options, comparative outcomes and associated complications. However, no individual recommendations concerning each specific sling system or data showing one sling is superior to another is available.

In addition, no guidelines concerning the ideal timing of surgical treatment are available. In general, surgical treatment should be offered if the incontinence status is stable despite intensive conservative treatment and on patients' demand.

Adjustable Sling Systems

Adjustable sling systems are positioned suburethrally on top of the bulbospongiosus muscle by a retropubic or transobturator approach. In these types of slings, postoperatively tension can be adjusted. Available devices are (alphabetical order): Argus classic, Argus T, ATOMS, Remeex.

In general, outcome is comparable for all adjustable sling systems (Table 4.1). However, there a differences in complications and adjustment techniques as well as invasiveness.

The risk of erosion seems to be linked to the degree of compression of the urethra and to infections. De novo urgency seems to be associated with mild postoperative obstruction.

Compared to retrourethral slings postoperative pain is more common after implantation of adjustable sling systems. Early postoperative

R.M. Bauer, M.D. (✉)
Department of Urology, Ludwig-Maximilians-University, München, Klinikum Großhadern, Marchioninistr. 15, Munich 81377, Germany
e-mail: ricarda.bauer@med.uni-muenchen.de

Table 4.1 Outcome of adjustable sling systems (no studies included reporting only salvage cases)

Publication	Type of sling	Number of patients	Mean/median follow-up (months)	Definition of success	Success rate (%)	Improved (%)	Explantation rate (%)
Hoda et al.	ATOMS	99	18	0 pads/day and <10 ml in 24 h pad test	63	29	4.0
Seweryn et al.	ATOMS	38	17	0–1 pad/day and <15 ml in 24 h pad test	60.5	23.7	15.8
Bochove-Overgaauw et al.	Argus classic	95	27	Dry or improved	72 (0 pads: 40 %)	18	11
Dalpiaz et al.	Argus classic	29	35	0–1 small safety pad/day	17	Not provided	35
Hübner et al.	Argus classic	101	25	≤1 ml in 20 min pad test	79.2	Not provided	15.8
Romano et al.	Argus classic	48	45	0 pads/day	66	13	10.4
Bauer et al.	ArgusT	42	28.8	0–5 ml in 24 h pad test	61.9	26.2	11.9 % (including failed patients)
Sousa-Escandon et al.	Remeex	51	32	≤1 pad/day	64.7	19.6	5.9
	Remeex						

pain is very common and even persistent pain can occur in up to 5 % of the patients.

Mode of Action

Permanent increase of urethral resistance 10–15 cm H_2O to support basis continence.

Argus Classic/ArgusT

The Argus system (Promedon, Argentina) consists of a radiopaque cushioned system with a silicone foam pad for soft compression of the bulbar urethra. Two silicone columns formed by multiple conical elements are attached to the silicone foam and allow system readjustment while two radiopaque silicone washers allow regulation of the desired tension (Fig. 4.1a, b). During implantation measurement of the retrograde leak point pressure (RLPP) is recommended. During intraoperative tensioning the silicone arms are tensioned through the washers until a RLPP of pre-adjustment RLPP + 10 cm H_2O is achieved (recommended maximum intraoperative RLPP 40 cm H_2O).

The Argus sling can be implanted via a retropubic (Argus classic—Fig. 4.2) or a transobturatoric (ArgusT—Fig. 4.3) approach.

For readjustment the suprapubic incision (Argus classic) respectively the right and left inguinal incisions (ArgusT) have to be re-opened under local or general anesthesia to explore the washers to increase or decrease the tension.

For the Argus classic several published studies with a mean follow-up period of up to 45 months are available. Reported cure rates are 17–79 %.

In 48 patients with mild-to-moderate SUI and a mean follow-up of 45 months (range 36–54 months), a dry rate of 66 % was achieved [7]. Another study evaluated 101 patients with moderate to severe SUI. After a mean follow-up of 2.1 years (range 0.1–4.5 years) a dry rate of 79.2 % (pad test of 0–1 g) was reported [8]. A retrospective study including 95 patients with severe SUI showed success rates (cured + improved) of 72 % and a dry rate of 40 % (0 pads) in a median follow-up of 27 months (range 14–57 months) [9].

Readjustments are required in approximately one third of the patients.

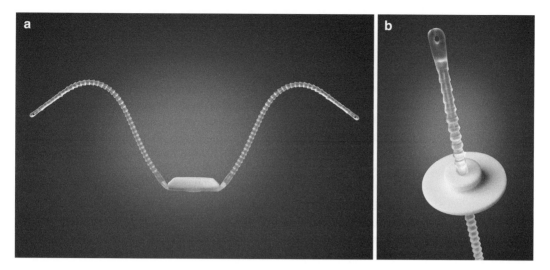

Fig. 4.1 (**a**) Argus system (with permission of Promedon, Argentina; copyright Promedon). (**b**) Argus Washer (with permission of Promedon, Argentina; copyright Promedon)

Fig. 4.2 Argus classic (with permission of Promedon, Argentina; copyright Promedon)

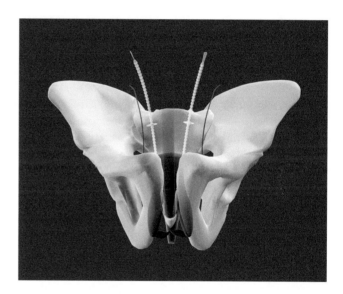

Fig. 4.3 Argus T (with permission of Promedon, Argentina; copyright Promedon)

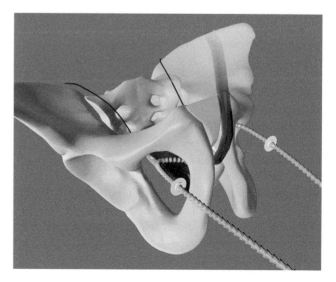

Data concerning irradiated patients are controversial showing equal [8, 10] or lower success rates [9] compared to non-irradiated patients. In addition, one study showed reduced efficacy in patients after treatment for urethral strictures or bladder neck stenosis before sling implantation [9]. Other studies showed no difference or did not evaluate these patients in detail.

Reported intraoperative complications of the Argus classic are bladder injuries (up to 10 %).

Main postoperative complications in a mean follow-up period of up to 45 months are: infections (up to 7 %), significant postoperative perineal pain (up to 27 %), urethral or bladder erosion (up to 13 %), de novo urgency (up to 14 %), retention (up to 35 %), suprapubic extrusion of the columns (up to 7 %), system dislocation (up to 7 %), and explantation of the system (up to 35 %) due to complications (e.g., infection, erosion, pain) [7–10]. In the early postoperative period urinary retention can occur (up to 35 %). Moderate adjustment of the sling during implantation (recommended maximum intraoperative retrograde leak point pressure <40 cm H_2O) seems to reduce the complication rate especially of postoperative retention and sling erosion [8].

Detailed information concerning late postoperative complications is rare. In up to 3 % persistent pain occurs and there is one reported case of explantation after several months due to persistent pain [10]. In general, for the first generation of the Argus classic more complications are reported [10].

The implantation technique of the ArgusT was first published in 2004 including one case report [11]. Until now, only one study with a mean follow-up of 28.8 months including 42 patients is published [3]. Dry rate with a pad test of 0–5 g/24 h was 61.9 %. 26.2 % of the patients had a reduction of incontinence of at least 50 % and five patients failed. In all patients the ArgusT was explanted and an artificial sphincter (AMS 800, American Medical Systems, USA) was successfully implanted. Subgroup analysis showed no difference in outcome of patients with additional radiotherapy, on patients with preoperative urine loss <500 g/24 h and >500 g/24 h and in patients with and without anti-incontinence pretreatment. In addition, type of prostate surgery, age, and BMI had also no impact on outcome.

Median adjustment rate was 1.7.

There were no intraoperative complications or postoperative urinary retention reported.

The following postoperative complications occurred: urinary tract infection (2.4 %), perineal wound infection (2.4 %), suprapubic wound infection (4.8 %), postoperative analgesics for >3 months (16.7 %), postoperative urgency (7.1 %), explantation due to persistent pain (4.8 %).

In general, the results of the Argus T seem to be comparable with the Argus classic. However, in contrast to the Argus classic, in the Argus T postoperative pain and persistent pain seems to be higher.

ATOMS

The ATOMS system (A.M.I., Austria) consists of an adjustable cushion fixed with monofilament polypropylene mesh arms around the Ramus inferior of the Os pubis (Fig. 4.4). The mesh arms establish a 4-point fixation. A titanium port for adjustment of the cushion volume is integrated and placed in the left symphysis (inguinal port—Fig. 4.5) or scrotal region (scrotal port—Fig. 4.6). The sling is implanted via a transobturator approach using a perineal single-incision. Compression of the bulbar urethra is achieved via the adjustable cushion.

For the ATOMS system, two studies are published. In both studies the ATOMS with perineal port was evaluated.

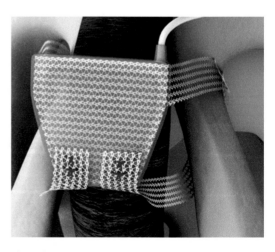

Fig. 4.4 Position of ATOMS (with permission of AMI, Austria; copyright AMI)

Fig. 4.5 ATOMS with inguinal port (with permission of AMI, Austria; copyright AMI)

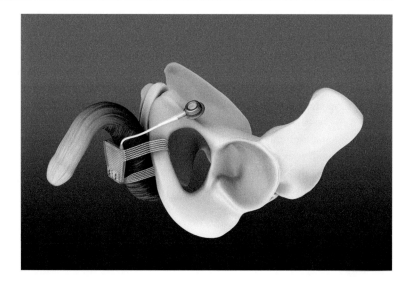

Fig. 4.6 ATOMS with scrotal port (with permission of AMI, Austria; copyright AMI)

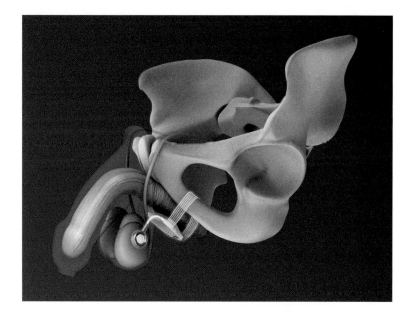

The first study evaluated 38 patients with a mean urine loss of 747 ml in the 24-h pad test (230–1600 ml) and a mean follow-up of 16.9 months (range 13–21 months) [12]. 60.5 % of the patients were considered dry (0–1 pads and less than 15 ml in the 24-h pad test) and 23.7 % improved (more than one pad and 16 to 100 ml in the 24-h pad test). In 15.8 % of the patients implantation failed (more than two pads daily or more than 100 ml in the 24-h pad test). Mean number of adjustments was 3.97 (range 0–9).

The second study evaluated 99 patients with a mean urine loss of 681 ml in the 24-h pad test [13]. After a mean follow-up of 17.8 months (range 12–33 months) 63 % of the patients were considered dry (0 pads and <10 ml in 24-h pad test) and 29 % were improved (daily pad use reduced by >50 % or patients needed 1–2 pads/24 h and 10–40 ml in 24-h pad test). 8 % of the patients failed. Mean number of adjustments was 3.8 (range 1–6). For every adjustment, 2 ml saline solution was added to the cushion via the port.

No intraoperative complications are published.

Reported postoperative complications are the following: transient perineal or scrotal pain/dysesthesia (up to 68.7 %), early port infections leading to explantation (up to 10.5 %), retention (up to 3 %), explantation due to persistent pain (up to 3 %) and urethral erosion (up to 3 %).

Patients with previous radiotherapy or previous surgery for incontinence show comparable results to non-irradiated/non-pretreated patients without a higher incidence of complications.

The impact of age, comorbidities on outcome or complications is not evaluated.

Remeex

The Remeex system (Neomedic, Spain) consists of a mesh connected via two monofilament traction threads to a suprapubic mechanical regulator and is positioned under the bulbar urethra (Fig. 4.7). The system is implanted via a retropubic approach. The regulation part—the so-called "varitensor"—is a permanent implant ($1 \times 1 \times 2.5$ cm cubic device with internal never-ending axis to wind the traction threads) subcutaneously over the abdominal rectum fascia above the pubis. Adjustment is conducted via an external manipulator starting on day 1 after implantation which stays in place after implantation. The external manipulator is removed after first adjustment.

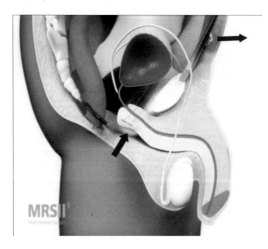

Fig. 4.7 Remeex (with permission of Neomedic, Spain, copyright Neomedic)

Subsequent adjustments are performed under local anesthesia via the rejoined external manipulator to the varitensor.

There are two published studies; however, one of them is only reporting preliminary results of six patients [14]. In a multicentric European Study 51 men with mild-to-severe SUI were treated with the Remeex [15]. The average follow-up was 32 months (range 16–50 months). 64.7 % of the patients were considered cured (no pads: 75.8 %; small pads or sanitary napkins for security reasons but normally dry: 24.2 %) and 19.6 % were improved. In 15.7 % of the patients the implantation failed.

90 % of the patients were adjusted during the early postoperative period; 86 % required a second adjustment between 1 to 4 months after implantation, and 33 % required more than two adjustments.

The only reported intraoperative complication is bladder perforation (up to 10 %).

Reported postoperative complications are transient perineal discomfort or pain in the majority of the patients. In addition, removal of the device (6 %) due to infections of the varitensor or due to urethral erosion is reported. During adjustment a rupture of the monofilament traction threads can occur. In addition, depending on degree of compression residual urine can occur.

The impact of age, comorbidities, or previous radiotherapy on outcome or complications is not evaluated.

Advantages and Disadvantages of Adjustable Sling Systems

Postoperative adjustment is possible—even after years. Tension can be adjusted to patients' increased postoperative physical activity. Good results are also in severe PPI and irradiated patients possible.

Adjustable sling systems are associated with overall higher complication and explantation rates in comparison to fixed male slings.

Outcome in patients after treatment for urethral strictures or bladder neck stenosis seems to be decreased.

Treatment after Failed Adjustable Sling System

If the continence status is not improved by adjustment salvage treatment should be considered if the patients ask for further improvement.

In general, AUS implantation is the salvage treatment of choice. Several studies showed AUS implantation after failed Argus sling and ATOMS is still possible without specific problems and shows good results without increased complication rate [8, 13, 16]. No data exist concerning salvage treatment after failed Remeex sling implantation. However, data should be comparable to Argus and ATOMS. The adjustable sling systems (especially the non-mesh parts—explantation of the mesh parts can result in damage of the collateral tissue especially the urethra) should be explantated before AUS explantation.

If there is a damage or slippage of the sling system exchange of the system can be considered. In addition, there is one study reporting the implantation of an AdVance sling after failed adjustable sling systems [17]. However, no detailed analysis of this subgroup is available. In general, before considering the implantation of a retrourethral sling after failed adjustable sling system a proper evaluation of the residual sphincter function and mobility of the posterior urethra is necessary. However, implantation of an AdVance sling as salvage treatment salvage treatment cannot be widely recommended and should only be performed in highly selected patients and by an extremely experienced surgeon.

Fixed Male Slings

Fixed male slings can be divided into two types:

- Retrourethral slings.
- Fixed compressive slings.

Mode of Action

The hypothesized mechanism is not thoroughly understood.

The mode of action of the retrourethral slings seems to be multifactorial:

- Correction of postoperative hypermobility of the posterior urethra.
- Increased length of functional urethra.
- Venous sealing effect.

The mode of action of fixed compressive slings may result from a combination of urethral compression with subsequent permanent increase of urethral resistance and angulation.

Retrourethral Slings

Worldwide, the AdVance sling (American Medical Systems, USA) is the most commonly used sling and the most evaluated sling with a couple of published studies—mainly single-center studies.

The AdVance sling is a retrourethral sling (Fig. 4.8). It consists of a polypropylene mesh and is positioned under the membranous urethra via a transobturatoric approach (Fig. 4.9).

For the correct placement of the sling dissection of the centrum tendineum is necessary. Here the sling is fixed on the bulb and thereafter adjusted. It is postulated that due to intraoperative adjustment the lax and descended supporting structures of the posterior urethra and sphincter region after prostate surgery are relocated into the former pre-prostatectomy position (Figs. 4.10a, b) [19, 20]. Several urodynamic studies suggest that the AdVance sling does not cause any obstruction to the urethra [20–22].

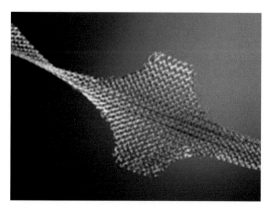

Fig. 4.8 AdVance sling (with permission of American Medical Systems, USA; copyright AMS)

Fig. 4.9 Position of
AdVance sling (with
permission of Elsevier [18])

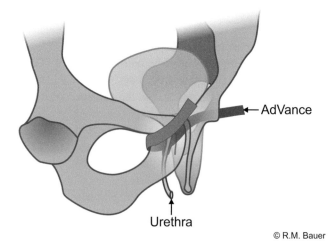

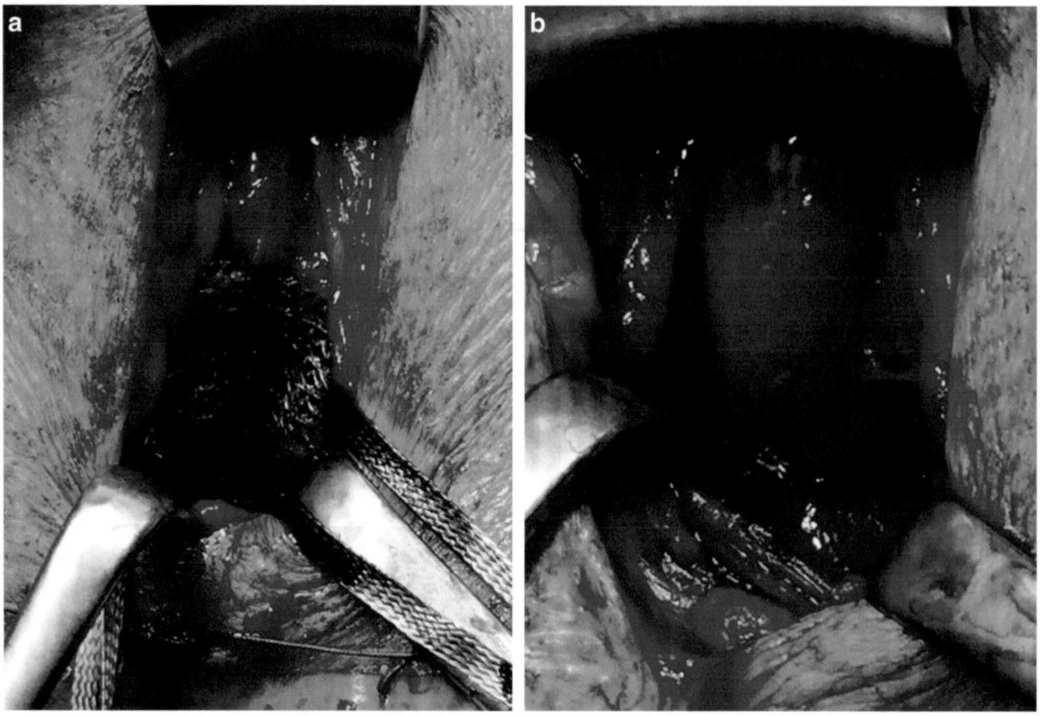

Fig. 4.10 (**a**) AdVance sling before adjustment. (**b**) AdVance sling after adjustment

For the AdVance sling cure rates of 9–63 % with a follow-up of up to 40 months are published [17, 23–30]. However, efficacy rates are difficult to compare due to heterogeneous definition for cure varying from 0 to 1 pad/day or different amounts of daily urine loss in pad tests (1-h pad test or 24-h pad test).

Two prospective studies with a 3 year follow-up including one multicentre study are available.

The multicentre study included 156 patients and reports a cure rate of 53 % (no pad or one security pad) and a success rate of 77 % (reduction of daily pad usage ≥50 %) [29]. No worsening over time occurred.

The second study included 30 patients and reported a cure rate of 60 % (no pad usage or one security pad) and a success rate of 73 % (reduction of daily pad usage ≥50 %) [28].

There are several risk factors for failure under discussion. Incontinence severity and residual sphincter function including ability to close the sphincter completely and functional sphincter lengths (≥ 1 cm) seem to have a positive effect on efficacy [19, 27, 29, 31, 32]. A Valsalva leak-point pressure of >100 cm H_2O, representing a good residual sphincter function and a lower degree of incontinence, is associated with better efficacy [33].

Surgery for urethral stenosis or anastomotic stricture between prostatectomy and sling implantation is significantly associated with lower dry rates [27].

In irradiated patients, the AdVance sling shows reduced treatment success with dry rates between 18 and 53 % [29, 34–36].

Previous surgical treatment may affect negatively the efficacy, especially if scarring of the surrounding tissue of the bulb occurred [28, 29]. However, there is one study reporting the outcome of AdVance sling implantation in 19 patients with recurrent stress incontinence after implantation of an artificial sphincter [37]. In all patients etiology of the recurrent stress incontinence was urethral atrophy. In all patients the AdVance sling was implanted in addition to the artificial sphincter. After a mean follow-up of 13 months 79 % were dry using no pads and 21 % were improved using one pad per day. 53 % of the dry patients were dry without reactivation of the artificial sphincter and 47 % maintained dry with a combination of the AdVance sling and the activated artificial sphincter. In these patients no intraoperative or postoperative complications (e.g., infection, retention, de novo urgency) occurred.

Patient age and body mass index seem to have no impact on outcome [28, 29].

In contrast, surgeon's experience (>25 AdVance sling implantation) may have a positive effect on outcome [32].

Severe complications including explantation or infection of the AdVance are rare.

The main postoperative complication is transient acute postoperative urinary retention (up to 21 %) requiring temporary recatheterization and mild postoperative perineal pain [17, 23–30, 38].

Two intraoperative injuries of the urethra are reported [38–40]. No further intraoperative complications are published.

Reported main early postoperative complications are transient acute postoperative urinary retention (up to 21 %) requiring temporary recatheterization, mild dysuria in 14 %, mild transient perineal or scrotal pain in 0–20 %, local wound infection 0.4 %, severe wound infection leading to sling explantation in 2.8 % ($n=1$), urinary infection with fever 0.4 % and perineal-adductor compartment haematoma under anticoagulation ($n=1$) [24, 27–29, 38, 41]. In addition, there is a report about one sling infection in an irradiated patient 5 months after second AdVance sling implantation resulting in explantation of both slings [42]. In general, explantation rate is very low with a very low number of reported cases in total (<10).

There are several studies dealing with late postoperative complications and were shown to be uncommon. However, the following late complications are reported: urinary retention for up to 5 months ($n=2$; 5.7 %), persistent retention due to sling slippage leading to sling incision ($n=1$; 0.4 %), persistent perineal pain ($n=1$; 0.4 %), significant adductor muscle pain ($n=2$; 1.7 %) and symphysitis ($n=1$; 0.4 %) leading to sling explantation—probably symphysitis was not induced by the sling [27–29, 38, 43].

The impact of age, comorbidities or previous radiotherapy on intraoperative or postoperative complications is not evaluated.

In end of 2010, the second generation—AdVanceXP– was introduced (Fig. 4.11). The AdVanceXP is not available in the USA (no FDA approval).

The AdVanceXP addresses several important issues:

- Anchors along the sling arms to reduce early failure due to sling loosening or slippage.
- A new needle shape for easier tunneling especially in larger or more obese patients.
- 4 cm longer sling arms.
- Tyvek liner protect sheaths on the sling arms to cover the anchors during implantation.

Three studies evaluating the efficacy and complications of the AdVance XP are published [23, 26, 44]. All three are comparative studies but not randomized. In general, efficacy of the AdVance XP seems to be comparable to the AdVance.

Fig. 4.11 AdVance XP
sling (with permission
of American Medical
Systems, USA;
copyright AMS)

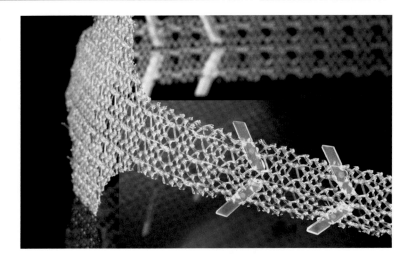

However, a new complication occurred: persistent residual urine.

In 110 patients treating with the AdVanceXP in a median follow-up of 16 months a cure rate of 59 % (no pad or one security pad) was reported [26]. Reported early postoperative complications are transient urinary retention (2 %) and perineal hematoma (<1 %). In addition some late complications occurred: persistent perineal pain (2 %) and de novo urgency 12 %. De novo urgency was successfully treated with anticholinergics.

In a second study 27 patients were included and the median follow-up was 26 months [44]. However no detailed outcome data was presented. Reported complications are transient urinary retention 15 %, perineal-scrotal pain 8 %, de novo urgency 8 % and perineal hematoma 3 %. De novo urgency was again successfully treated with anticholinergics. A risk factor analysis showed only amount of urine loss in the 24-h pad test with significant impact on outcome. There was no impact on outcome for age, body mass index, interval from prostatectomy to sling placement, quality of life score, radiotherapy, weak sphincter coaptation, adverse urodynamics and sling fixation.

In the third study 41 patients with a median follow-up of 25 months were included [23]. 65.9 % were cured (0 or one security pad). Median pad weight in the 24-h pad test was in all patients 8 g. A subgroup analysis showed better efficacy of the AdVanceXP in comparison to the AdVance in obese patients (body mass index 25.0–30.0). The following complications occurred: de novo urgency 2.4 %,

urinary tract infection 4.9 % and temporary elevated residual urine 7.3 %. In 5 % ($n=2$) persistent urinary retention occurred. In both patients one sling arm was resected after 3 months resulting in normal voiding without residual urine and without negative impact on continence. In both cases the presumed reason for persistent urinary retention was an intraoperative overtensioning of the sling during removal of the Tyvek liner protect sheaths. Therefore caution is recommended during removal of the protect sheaths.

Fixed Compressive Slings

There are two types of fixed compressive slings:

- Bone-anchored slings.
- Non-bone-anchored slings.

Bone-Anchored Slings

The InVance sling (American Medical Systems, USA) has become the most commonly utilized bone-anchored sling. The sling consists of a silicon-coated polyester sling positioned under the bulbar urethra via a perineal incision to achieve compression (Fig. 4.12). The mode of action results in compression to the bulbar urethra through placement of the mesh which is secured to both inferior ischiopubic rami by three titanium screws at each side. Commercialization of the InVance was stopped in mid-2014 by American Medical Systems and the sling is no longer available.

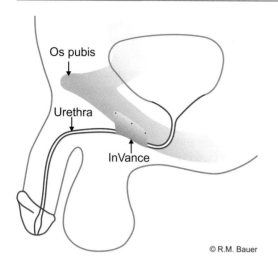

Os pubis

Urethra

InVance

© R.M. Bauer

Fig. 4.12 Position of InVance (with permission of Elsevier [18])

For the InVance sling data with a long follow-up period (up to 4 years) exist. In patients with mild-to-severe SUI pad free rates range from 36 to 65 % and improvement rates are 10–40 % [45–53]. Failure rates in irradiated patients are higher (up to 85 %) compared to non-irradiated patients [52, 53]. No intraoperative complications are reported. The main reported postoperative complication is perineal pain. It occurs in up to 76 % of the patients but usually resolves within 3 months. However, persistent pain is also reported and may require explantation of the sling [49, 54]. Additionally, residual urine occurs in up to 12 %. In most cases residual urine resolved by itself without further treatment. Urinary retention requiring loosening of the sling is rare [51]. Further reported complications are increased explantation due to infection (up to 15 %) and bone-anchor dislodgement (up to 5 %). De novo urgency or urge-incontinence mostly associated with mild postoperative obstruction was reported in up to 14 % [45, 49, 54]. However, in most cases it can be treated successfully with oral anti-muscarinics. Urethral erosion is rare. However in these cases sling explantation is necessary [54].

There are several studies dealing with late postoperative complications of the InVance in detail [48–50, 52, 54]. The following late complications are reported: persistent pain in up to 12 % of the patients requiring analgesic management

and bone-anchor dislodgment leading to explantation. In addition, sling explantation due to infection is reported with an average time between implantation and explantation of 99 days (35–163 days).

One study evaluated the impact of obesity (BMI ≥30) and previous bladder neck contracture on intraoperative or postoperative complications. These patients showed a 51.5 % respectively 81.5 % risk of having ≥1 complications [55]. In contrast, no study evaluated the impact of age or previous radiotherapy on intraoperative or postoperative complications.

Non-bone-anchored Fixed Compressive Slings

Three non-bone-anchored fixed compressive slings with published data are available:

- Virtue sling (Coloplast, Denmark).
- TOMS and I-stop TOMS (CL Medical, USA).
- Compressive inside-out transobturator sling (Gynemesh PS, Ethicon, USA).

All these slings are positioned on the bulbospongiosus muscle and are implanted via a transobturator approach.

For the Virtue sling, a fixed four-arm sling with two transobturator arms and two pre-pubic arms, two published studies are available. The first study including 22 patients is mainly dealing with the implantation technique including the evaluation of the retrograde leak point pressure before and during implantation and is not focusing on efficacy or postoperative complications. After implantation an increase of the leak point pressure was measured. No intraoperative complications occurred [56]. The second study, a multicentre study reports 1 year data of 98 patients with mild-to-severe PPI and in addition the data of 31 patients with a novel fixation mechanism to prevent postoperative loosing or slippage of the sling [57]. 15 % of the patients were cured (<1.3 g urine loss in the 24-h pad test) after 12 months and 41.9 % showed an improvement of ≥50 % in the pad weight. All reported complications were Clavien grade I: 12.2 % short-term genital paraesthesia, 14.3 % temporary perineal pain, 1 % scrotal hematoma, and

1 % urinary tract infection. No erosion or sling infection occurred within 12 months. In the 31 patients with additional fixation of the sling arms the outcome was significantly better. After 12 months cure rate was 46 and 79.2 % improved. Complications were comparable to the non-fixation group. All complications were Clavien grade I: 19.4 % short-term genital paraesthesia and 12.9 % temporary perineal pain. In the patients with unfixed sling there was a progressive reduction in efficacy over the first year after implantation. Higher degree of PPI seems to have no negative impact on efficacy.

In both published studies the impact of previous radiotherapy on outcome or complications is not evaluated.

For the TOMS (a transobturatoric two-armed sling) two studies with a follow-up to 1 year [58, 59] and for I-stop TOMS (a transobturatoric four-armed sling) two studies with a follow-up up to 2 years are available [60, 61]. The slings can be implanted in an outside-in-technique as well as an inside-out-technique.

In patients with mild-to-moderate PPI a cure rate of 55.0 % (TOMS) respectively 50.0 % (I-stop TOMS) was achieved after 1 year with an improvement rate of 32.5 % resp. 46.1 %. After 2 years cure rate of the I-stop TOMS was in 21 evaluated patients 47.6 % and improvement rate was 42.8 %. In up to 4 % of the patients an intraoperative wounding of the corpus cavernosum is reported. Postoperatively, 8.7 % of the patients showed a hematoma. Wound infection within the first postoperative months is reported in 2 %. Postoperative urinary retention occurred in 1.1 % and urinary infections in up to 2.7 % of the patients. Perineal pain was very rare with maximum pain immediate postoperatively (2.7 ± 1.9 in the visual analog scale). At the 3 months follow-up 18.4 % of the patients had still a low stream or difficulties with voiding, decreasing to 13 % after 12 months.

The impact of previous radiotherapy on outcome or complications is not evaluated.

For the compressive inside-out transobturator sling by Gynemesh PS one published study including 173 patients is available [62]. After a median follow-up of 24 months (range: 12–60 month), 49 % of the patients were cured (no pad usage), 35 % improved (number of pads per day reduced by ≥ 50 % and two or fewer pads), and 16 % failed. Patient after previous radiotherapy showed a significant lower success rate. In addition a history of bladder neck stenosis resp. anastomosis stricture as well as obesity were independent risk factors of failure. No intraoperative complications occurred. There was only one suspected intraoperative bladder perforation in an irradiated patient. The angle of the guide insertion was reoriented and ureteroscopy evaluation was without any finding. Reported early postoperative complications are: urinary retention in 15 %, perineal/scrotal hematoma in 9 %, perineal pain up to 23 % and sling infection in 7.7 % (managed conservatively without sling explantation). Reported late postoperative complications are persistent pain in up to 5 % of the patients. At the follow-up visits at 1 and 2 years after implantation, four patients (3 %) respectively one patient (1 %) still suffered from pain. No patient reported persistent pain after 3 years. No urethral erosion or mesh removal/loosening were seen.

Advantages and Disadvantages of Fixed Male Slings

The AdVance sling is the treatment with highest number of published studies and highest number of treated patients. Best results can be achieved in patients with good residual sphincter function with mild-to-moderate PPI and mobile posterior urethra.

Complications in fixed slings are rare and mainly mild.

No postoperative adjustment is possible.

Irradiated patients, patients with severe PPI or with sphincter defect and patients after treatment for urethral strictures or bladder neck/anastomosis stenosis show reduced success rates.

Treatment after Failed Fixed Male Slings

After failed Invance sling implantation of an artificial sphincter is possible and shows good results. For implantation of an artificial sphincter the sling has to be divided at its mid-portion. In the short term (follow-up 14.2 months) outcome and complication is comparable to virgin patients [63].

Two studies are dealing with salvage therapy after failed AdVance sling in detail.

One study compared efficacy and safety of the implantation of an artificial sphincter after failed AdVance sling with primary sphincter implantation [64]. In 29 patients with failed AdVance sling an AUS was implanted via a perineal approach. In all cases, the cuff was placed distally to the sling around the intercrural bulbar urethra. After a follow-up of 20.4 months efficacy was comparable to primary AUS implantation with no increased complication rate.

Another study was evaluating the efficacy and safety of a second AdVance sling implantation after failed first AdVance sling in 35 patients [65]. After a mean follow-up of 16.6 months 34.5 % of the patients were cured (no pad use) and another 37.9 % were using one dry security pad. In one patient intraoperative urethral injury occurred. In this patient sling placement was continued and a cystourethrography was performed on day 6 before catheter removal. Postoperative urinary retention occurred in 23.6 % but was in all patients only temporary. No infection, erosion or persistent pain occurred.

No data exist concerning salvage treatment after failed implantation of a Virtue sling, a TOMS, an I-stop TOMS or the compressive inside-out transobturator sling. However, data should be comparable to other fixed male slings.

Patient Selection

There is currently no universally accepted standard by which patients are evaluated for persistent PPI nor stratified into receiving an adjustable or fixed male sling. In addition, comparative studies

for the different sling types are missing and no standardized definition for "dry" or "success" after sling implantation exists. Therefore, it is not possible to compare directly reported outcomes and complications and it is not possible to identify one sling procedure as superior over another.

In general, the selection of the treatment should be based on contraindications (Table 4.2). However, there is a wide overlap of the different surgical options.

The ideal population for the fixed slings and especially the AdVance/AdVanceXP sling is still under discussion. Some urologist uses the daily pad usage (mainly 2–3 pads/day) or the urine loss in a pad tests (often below 200 ml in 24 h). However, this is not very accurate and severity of incontinence is often under- or overestimated. Therefore, more objective criteria are necessary. Several studies showed that with the "repositioning test" a preoperative patient selection is possible [19, 31, 32]. The "repositioning test" is performed in lithotomy position with a cystoscope positioned distal to the membranous urethra. Gentle midperineal pressure is applied parallel to the anal canal and below the bulbar urethra for repositioning the membranous urethra. The test is positive if (1) the sphincter closes autonomously, reflex, concentrically and complete during repositioning of the membranous urethra and (2) if the functional urethra length = coaptive zone during additional active sphincter contraction (circumferential coaptation of the membranous urethra) is ≥1 cm.

In addition, patients with nocturinal incontinence, irradiated patients and patients with a history of bladder neck stenosis/anastomosis stricture seem to be poor candidates for any type of non-adjustable sling system [27, 29, 32–34].

Table 4.2 Preoperative patient selection

Fixed slings	Adjustable sling systems	AUS

• PPI I–II°
 • Mobile posterior urethra
 • Coaptive zone ≥1 cm
 • No PPI III°
 • No sphincter defect
 • Caveat:
  – Radiotherapy
  – History of bladder neck stenosis/anastomosis stricture
	• PPI II–III° (storage of urine still possible)
	 • AUS impossible or not accepted
	 • Irradiated patients: no decreased outcome
	 • Caveat:
	  – History of bladder neck stenosis/ anastomosis stricture
		• PPI II–III°
		 • Severe/complete sphincter defect
		 • Complete incontinence
		 • High psychological strain

Table 4.3 Treatment of persistent pain after sling implantation

Nociceptive pain	Neuropathic pain	Mixed pain
First line: Analgesics according to the WHO scheme • WHO stage I: non-opioid analgesics ± adjuvant • WHO stage II: weak opioids, add if necessary non-opioid analgesics ± adjuvant • WHO stage III: strong opioids, add if necessary non-opioid analgesics ± adjuvant *Second line*: Sling explantation	*First line*: • Stabbing pain: Anticonvulsants (e.g., gabapentin or pregabalin) • Burning pain: tricyclic antidepressants (e.g., amitriptyline) or retarded opioids (e.g., tramadol). *Second line*: Pudendal nerve block *Third line*: Sling explantation	*First line*: • Combination of treatment for neuropathic pain with non-opioid analgesics ± adjuvant *Second line*: Sling explantation

Management of Persistent Pain after Sling Implantation

Persistent pain can occur in up to 5 % of the patients especially after implantation of a transobturatoric adjustable sling system.

Potential explanations may be the higher trauma and compression to the Pudendus and Obturatorius nerve and its branches.

The treatment of persistent pain is a huge challenge for urologists as well as patients.

After pain classification (nociceptive, neuropathic, mixed) and exclusion of an infection or erosion of the sling system, pain management should be started. In cases of nociceptive pain nonsteroidal antirheumatics, COX2-inhibitors or metamizole seems to be helpful; if necessary treatment escalation with a weak opioid is recommended. In cases of neuropathic pain Pregabalin, Gabapentin, tricyclic antidepressants (e.g., amitriptyline) or retarded opioids (e.g., tramadol) are effective. If not effective an interventional procedure should be performed (Table 4.3). Only in rare cases a sling explantation is necessary [66].

Conclusion

The treatment of post-prostatectomy stress urinary incontinence has evolved significantly over the past decades, with numerous improvements including various types of male sling systems.

Patients' demand for sling implantation is high and the opportunity to avoid using a mechanical device is preferable to undergoing a well-established procedure.

Male slings are nowadays widely used for the treatment of particularly mild-to-moderate PPI. However, there are no comparative studies. Therefore, it is not possible to compare directly reported outcomes and complications and it is not possible to identify one sling procedure as superior over another.

In general, surgical intervention should only be offered, if the incontinence status is stable and no further improvement of continence can be achieved with conservative treatment.

In the next future new variations and improvements to the existing male slings will be developed and further studies with long-term follow-up data will be available.

Patients with persistent PPI desiring sling implantation should be counseled as to reasonable expected outcomes as well as potential complications.

References

1. Berry JL. Evaluation of a new procedure for correction of postprostatectomy urinary incontinence. Bull N Y Acad Med. 1964;40:790–4.
2. Kaufman JJ. Surgical treatment of post-prostatectomy urinary incontinence: use of penile crura to compress the bulbous urethra. J Urol. 1972;107:293.
3. Schaeffer AJ, Clemens JQ, Ferrari M, et al. The male bulbourethral sling procedure for post-radical prostatectomy incontinence. J Urol. 1998;159:1510–5.

4. Kumar A, Litt ER, Ballert KN, et al. Artificial urinary sphincter versus male sling for post-prostatectomy incontinence--what do patients choose? J Urol. 2009;181:1231–5.
5. Abrams P, Cardozo L, Khoury S, et al. Incontinence - 4th international consultation on incontinence. Paris: Health Publication Ltd; 2009.
6. Lucas MG, Bosch RJ, Burkhard FC, et al. EAU guidelines on surgical treatment of urinary incontinence. Eur Urol. 2012;62:1118–29.
7. Romano SV, Metrebian SE, Vaz F, et al. Long-term results of a phase III multicentre trial of the adjustable male sling for treating urinary incontinence after prostatectomy: minimum 3 years. Actas Urol Esp. 2009;33:309–14.
8. Hubner WA, Gallistl H, Rutkowski M, et al. Adjustable bulbourethral male sling: experience after 101 cases of moderate-to-severe male stress urinary incontinence. BJU Int. 2011;107:777–82.
9. Bochove-Overgaauw DM, Schrier BP. An adjustable sling for the treatment of all degrees of male stress urinary incontinence: retrospective evaluation of efficacy and complications after a minimal followup of 14 months. J Urol. 2011;185:1363–8.
10. Dalpiaz O, Knopf HJ, Orth S, et al. Mid-term complications after placement of the male adjustable suburethral sling: a single center experience. J Urol. 2011;186:604–9.
11. Palma PC, Dambros M, Thiel M, et al. Readjustable transobturator sling: a novel sling procedure for male urinary incontinence. Urol Int. 2004;73:354–6.
12. Seweryn J, Bauer W, Ponholzer A, et al. Initial experience and results with a new adjustable transobturator male system for the treatment of stress urinary incontinence. J Urol. 2012;187:956–61.
13. Hoda MR, Primus G, Fischereder K, et al. Early results of a European multicentre experience with a new self-anchoring adjustable transobturator system for treatment of stress urinary incontinence in men. BJU Int. 2013;111:296–303.
14. Sousa-Escandon A, Rodriguez Gomez JI, Uribarri Gonzalez C, et al. Externally readjustable sling for treatment of male stress urinary incontinence: points of technique and preliminary results. J Endourol. 2004;18:113–8.
15. Sousa-Escandon A, Cabrera J, Mantovani F, et al. Adjustable suburethral sling (male remeex system) in the treatment of male stress urinary incontinence: a multicentric European study. Eur Urol. 2007;52:1473–9.
16. Bauer RM, Rutkowski M, Kretschmer A, et al. Efficacy and complications of the adjustable sling system ArgusT for male incontinence: results of a prospective 2-center study. Urology. 2015;85:316–20.
17. Bauer RM, Soljanik I, Fullhase C, et al. Mid-term results for the retroluminar transobturator sling suspension for stress urinary incontinence after prostatectomy. BJU Int. 2011;108:94–8.
18. Bauer RM, Bastian PJ, Gozzi C, et al. Postprostatectomy incontinence: all about diagnosis and management. Eur Urol. 2009;55:322–33.
19. Rehder P, Freiin Von Gleissenthall G, Pichler R, et al. The treatment of postprostatectomy incontinence with the retroluminal transobturator repositioning sling (Advance): lessons learnt from accumulative experience. Arch Esp Urol. 2009;62:860–70.
20. Rehder P, Gozzi C. Transobturator sling suspension for male urinary incontinence including post-radical prostatectomy. Eur Urol. 2007;52:860–6.
21. Davies TO, Bepple JL, Mccammon KA. Urodynamic changes and initial results of the AdVance male sling. Urology. 2009;74:354–7.
22. Soljanik I, Becker AJ, Stief CG, et al. Urodynamic parameters after retrourethral transobturator male sling and their influence on outcome. Urology. 2011;78:708–12.
23. Bauer RM, Kretschmer A, Stief CG, et al. AdVance and AdVance XP slings for the treatment of postprostatectomy incontinence. World J Urol. 2015;33:145–50.
24. Berger AP, Strasak A, Seitz C, et al. Single institution experience with the transobturator sling suspension system AdVance(R) in the treatment of male urinary incontinence: mid-term results. Int Braz J Urol. 2011;37:488–94.
25. Cornel EB, Elzevier HW, Putter H. Can advance transobturator sling suspension cure male urinary postoperative stress incontinence? J Urol. 2010;183:1459–63.
26. Cornu JN, Batista Da Costa J, Henry N, et al. Comparative study of AdVance and AdVanceXP male slings in a tertiary reference center. Eur Urol. 2014;65:502–4.
27. Cornu JN, Sebe P, Ciofu C, et al. Mid-term evaluation of the transobturator male sling for post-prostatectomy incontinence: focus on prognostic factors. BJU Int. 2011;108:236–40.
28. Kowalik CG, Delong JM, Mourtzinos AP. The advance transobturator male sling for post-prostatectomy incontinence: subjective and objective outcomes with 3 years follow up. Neurourol Urodyn. 2015;34:251–4.
29. Rehder P, Haab F, Cornu JN, et al. Treatment of post-prostatectomy male urinary incontinence with the transobturator retroluminal repositioning sling suspension: 3-year follow-up. Eur Urol. 2012;62:140–5.
30. Suskind AM, Bernstein B, Murphy-Setzko M. Patient-perceived outcomes of the AdVance sling up to 40 months post procedure. Neurourol Urodyn. 2011;30:1267–70.
31. Bauer RM, Gozzi C, Roosen A, et al. Impact of the 'repositioning test' on postoperative outcome of retroluminar transobturator male sling implantation. Urol Int. 2013;90:334–8.
32. Soljanik I, Gozzi C, Becker AJ, et al. Risk factors of treatment failure after retrourethral transobturator male sling. World J Urol. 2012;30:201–6.
33. Barnard J, Van Rij S, Westenberg AM. A Valsalva leak-point pressure of >100 cmH$_2$O is associated with greater success in AdVance sling placement for the

treatment of post-prostatectomy urinary incontinence. BJU Int. 2014;114 Suppl 1:34–7.

34. Bauer RM, Soljanik I, Fullhase C, et al. Results of the AdVance transobturator male sling after radical prostatectomy and adjuvant radiotherapy. Urology. 2011;77:474–9.

35. Torrey R, Rajeshuni N, Ruel N, et al. Radiation history affects continence outcomes after advance transobturator sling placement in patients with post-prostatectomy incontinence. Urology. 2013;82:713–7.

36. Zuckerman JM, Tisdale B, Mccammon K. AdVance male sling in irradiated patients with stress urinary incontinence. Can J Urol. 2011;18:6013–7.

37. Christine B, Knoll LD. Treatment of recurrent urinary incontinence after artificial urinary sphincter placement using the AdVance male sling. Urology. 2010;76:1321–4.

38. Bauer RM, Mayer ME, May F, et al. Complications of the AdVance transobturator male sling in the treatment of male stress urinary incontinence. Urology. 2010;75:1494–8.

39. Harris SE, Guralnick ML, O'connor RC. Urethral erosion of transobturator male sling. Urology. 2009;73(443):e419–20.

40. Rehder P. Re: Harris SE, Guralnick ML, O'Connor RC: Urethral erosion of transobturator male sling. (Urology 2009;73:443). Urology. 2009;73:449–50. author reply 450.

41. Kruck S, Bedke J, Amend B, et al. Underestimated risk of bleeding after male transobturator sling procedure caused by early re-uptake of anticoagulation. Urol Int. 2011;86:242–4.

42. Weinberger JM, Purohit RS, Blaivas JG. Mesh infection of a male sling. J Urol. 2013;190:1054–5.

43. Gill BC, Swartz MA, Klein JB, et al. Patient perceived effectiveness of a new male sling as treatment for post-prostatectomy incontinence. J Urol. 2010;183:247–52.

44. Collado Serra A, Resel Folkersma L, Dominguez-Escrig JL, et al. AdVance/AdVance XP transobturator male slings: preoperative degree of incontinence as predictor of surgical outcome. Urology. 2013;81:1034–9.

45. Athanasopoulos A, Konstantinopoulos A, Mcguire E. Efficacy of the InVance male sling in treating stress urinary incontinence: a three-year experience from a single centre. Urol Int. 2010;85:436–42.

46. Carmel M, Hage B, Hanna S, et al. Long-term efficacy of the bone-anchored male sling for moderate and severe stress urinary incontinence. BJU Int. 2010;106:1012–6.

47. Castle EP, Andrews PE, Itano N, et al. The male sling for post-prostatectomy incontinence: mean followup of 18 months. J Urol. 2005;173:1657–60.

48. Comiter CV. The male perineal sling: intermediate-term results. Neurourol Urodyn. 2005;24:648–53.

49. Fassi-Fehri H, Badet L, Cherass A, et al. Efficacy of the InVance male sling in men with stress urinary incontinence. Eur Urol. 2007;51:498–503.

50. Gallagher BL, Dwyer NT, Gaynor-Krupnick DM, et al. Objective and quality-of-life outcomes with bone-anchored male bulbourethral sling. Urology. 2007;69:1090–4.

51. Giberti C, Gallo F, Schenone M, et al. The bone-anchor sub-urethral sling for the treatment of iatrogenic male incontinence: subjective and objective assessment after 41 months of mean follow-up. World J Urol. 2008;26:173–8.

52. Giberti C, Gallo F, Schenone M, et al. The bone anchor suburethral synthetic sling for iatrogenic male incontinence: critical evaluation at a mean 3-year followup. J Urol. 2009;181:2204–8.

53. Guimaraes M, Oliveira R, Pinto R, et al. Intermediate-term results, up to 4 years, of a bone-anchored male perineal sling for treating male stress urinary incontinence after prostate surgery. BJU Int. 2009;103:500–4.

54. Fischer MC, Huckabay C, Nitti VW. The male perineal sling: assessment and prediction of outcome. J Urol. 2007;177:1414–8.

55. Styn NR, Mcguire EJ, Latini JM. Bone-anchored sling for male stress urinary incontinence: assessment of complications. Urology. 2011;77:469–73.

56. Comiter CV, Nitti V, Elliot C, et al. A new quadratic sling for male stress incontinence: retrograde leak point pressure as a measure of urethral resistance. J Urol. 2012;187:563–8.

57. Comiter CV, Rhee EY, Tu LM, et al. The virtue sling-a new quadratic sling for postprostatectomy incontinence--results of a multinational clinical trial. Urology. 2014;84:433–8.

58. Grise P, Geraud M, Lienhart J, et al. Transobturator male sling TOMS for the treatment of stress post-prostatectomy incontinence, initial experience and results with one year's experience. Int Braz J Urol. 2009;35:706–13. discussion 714-705.

59. Yiou R, Loche CM, Lingombet O, et al. Evaluation of urinary symptoms in patients with post-prostatectomy urinary incontinence treated with the male sling TOMS. Neurourol Urodyn. 2015;34:12–7.

60. Drai J, Caremel R, Riou J, et al. The two-year outcome of the I-Stop TOMS transobturator sling in the treatment of male stress urinary incontinence in a single centre and prediction of outcome. Prog Urol. 2013;23:1494–9.

61. Grise P, Vautherin R, Njinou-Ngninkeu B, et al. I-STOP TOMS transobturator male sling, a minimally invasive treatment for post-prostatectomy incontinence: continence improvement and tolerability. Urology. 2012;79:458–63.

62. Leruth J, Waltregny D, De Leval J. The inside-out transobturator male sling for the surgical treatment of stress urinary incontinence after radical prostatectomy: midterm results of a single-center prospective study. Eur Urol. 2012;61:608–15.

63. Fisher MB, Aggarwal N, Vuruskan H, et al. Efficacy of artificial urinary sphincter implantation after failed bone-anchored male sling for postprostatectomy incontinence. Urology. 2007;70:942–4.

64. Lentz AC, Peterson AC, Webster GD. Outcomes following artificial sphincter implantation after prior unsuccessful male sling. J Urol. 2012;187:2149–53.

65. Soljanik I, Becker AJ, Stief CG, et al. Repeat retrourethral transobturator sling in the management of recurrent postprostatectomy stress urinary incontinence after failed first male sling. Eur Urol. 2010;58:767–72.

66. Bauer RM, Hubner W, Knopf HJ, et al. [Adjustable transobturatoric sling system in men: diagnosis and therapy recommendations to persistent pain]. Urologe A. 2014;53:1175–80.

Artificial Urinary Sphincter: Patient Selection and Surgical Technique

Joseph J. Pariser, Andrew J. Cohen,
Alexandre M. Rosen, and Gregory T. Bales

Background and Device

The AUS has long been considered the gold standard for post-prostatectomy incontinence (PPI) since its development by Dr. Scott in 1973 [1]. A far more primitive device was introduced by Dr. Foley in 1947, which included an external compression device on the urethra and a manual pump [2]. The only currently available model of the artificial urinary sphincter is the AMS 800 three-piece sphincter, which is shown in Fig. 5.1. The main components of the device are the pressure regulating balloon (also sometimes referred to as the reservoir), inflatable cuff and the control pump. The system is filled with isotonic fluid and functions by relying on the pressure maintained by the reservoir and a valve lockout system. At rest, the device remains in the "activated" position, which indicates that the cuff is inflated and occluding the urethra. When the control pump is

J.J. Pariser, M.D. (✉) • A.J. Cohen, M.D.
G.T. Bales, M.D.
Section of Urology, University of Chicago Medicine,
5841 S. Maryland Ave. MC 6038, Chicago, IL 60637,
USA
e-mail: Joseph.Pariser@uchospitals.edu;
Andrew.Cohen@uchospitals.edu;
gbales@surgery.bsd.uchicago.edu

A.M. Rosen, M.D.
Specialists in Urology, 955 10th Ave. North, Naples,
FL 34102, USA

squeezed, the fluid evacuates from the cuff and due to the pressure gradient, enters the reservoir. After roughly 90 s, the cuff automatically reinflates by fluid returning from the reservoir. It is possible to maintain the "deactivated" position by depressing a button located on the superior aspect of the control pump. When reactivating the pump by forcefully depressing the main portion of the pump, there is often a palpable click as the poppet valve unseats and the device is reactivated.

The AMS 800 is instilled with an antibiotic coating of InhibiZone, which contains minocycline and rifampin. Studies related to effectiveness have generally been in the setting of other genitourinary prosthetic surgery, specifically inflatable penile prosthesis (IPP). Carson showed a decreased risk of infection complications for IPP treated with InhibiZone compared to controls [3], which was corroborated in other studies [4]. However, studies specifically in AUS have not demonstrated an obvious benefit from the antibiotic coating in terms of infectious complications, though the coating is associated with increased costs [5]. Nonetheless, InhibiZone remains the standard antibiotic coating on AMS 800, though non-coated devices are available. When using antibiotic coated devices, they may be externally rinsed occasionally with fluid, but they should not be soaked in saline as this can dilute its concentration. Of note, the use of InhibiZone is contraindicated in patients with known allergy to tetracyclines or rifampin.

© Springer International Publishing Switzerland 2016
J.S. Sandhu (ed.), *Urinary Dysfunction in Prostate Cancer*, DOI 10.1007/978-3-319-23817-3_5

Fig. 5.1 AMS 800
artificial urinary
sphincter (courtesy of
AMS)

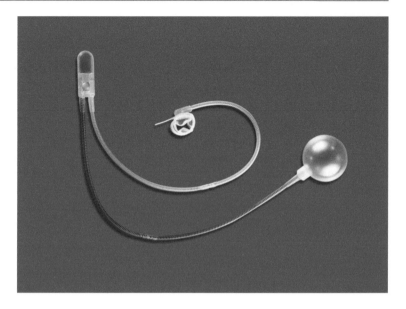

Additionally, InhibiZone is contraindicated for those patients with systemic lupus erythematosus as minocycline has been reported to exacerbate the disease [6].

Patient Selection

History and Physical Exam

When considering placement of the artificial urinary sphincter, a successful outcome begins in the clinic. While urologists have some surgical options for the treatment of incontinence, many patients are not appropriate candidates for one or more therapies. Estimates of incontinence after prostatectomy vary based on series as well as the definition of incontinence used, but multiple series report a 7–16 % incidence of some level of leakage [7–9]. Patients with other causes of stress incontinence are candidates for AUS, including those with spinal cord injuries and women with intrinsic sphincter deficiency.

A thorough urologic history is important to ascertain and should identify the cause of incontinence. The surgeon should be careful to elicit any other priorabdominopelvic surgeries that may complicate reservoir placement. The degree of incontinence, usually in terms of the numbers of pads used daily and the degree to which they are

soaked, should also be evaluated as alternative treatments are reasonable for less severe incontinence [10]. Some men with mild leakage may elect to undergo sling placement or injection of bulking agents. Of note, the number of pads alone has been thought to be unreliable as there is considerable variation in the amount of urine leakage tolerable by men before absorbent pads are changed. Some urologists, in an effort to be more accurate, may utilize other instruments, such as pad weight. In theSUFU Pad Test Study, Nitti et al. demonstrated that the subjective patient-perceived amount of leakage actually correlated well with the true amount of leakage by weighing pads over 24 h [11]. Utilizing newer technology, Pepper et al. demonstrated the feasibility and usefulness of a mobile app to document urinary incontinence symptoms [12]. Such an approach can be used as an alternative to the traditional bladder diary or patient recall. No matter the approach, understanding the degree of leakage with a patient preoperatively can help to realistically set expectations of dryness after any planned procedure.

Identifying those patients with primarily urge incontinence remains an important step before AUS placement as implantation of the device may exacerbate rather than relieve symptoms of urgency. As an elevated detrusor leak point pressure of over 40 cm water has been shown to be associated with upper tract deterioration [13, 14], increasing outflow resistance in the setting of a "hostile" bladder is a risk and may lead to renal deterioration. In the setting of prior radiotherapy, Gomha and Boone reported similar outcomes of AUS for post-prostatectomy incontinence compared to those without radiation though urinary urgency was notably high (44–47 %) in both groups [15]. Additionally, Ravier et al. reported similar functional outcomes but increased rate of major complications for AUS placement in patients with prior radiation [16]. A largemulti-center prospective study of 386 patients demonstrated that radiation, prior AUS erosion and history of urethral stent increased the risk of AUS explantation [17]. Taken in total, the risks and benefits should be carefully assessed before any surgical undertaking in these higher risk patients, though AUS placement certainly is feasible and usually met with excellent outcomes.

Understanding a patient's wishes and expectations is another critical preoperative step. Those with mild urinary incontinence may prefer to live with their symptoms rather than pursue AUS placement given its associated morbidity and risk. Additionally, other surgical procedures, such as sling placement or injection of bulking agents, may be viable alternative therapies for certain patients. Given that a significant portion of the psychosocial impact associated with stress urinary incontinence is related to the quantity of loss of urine [18], a reasonable nonsurgical option to prevent leakage is the use of an external Cunningham clamp, a device that has been shown to outperform other penile compression devices [19]. With an AUS, there is some concern about the need to manage a mechanical device in order to urinate, which is one advantage of using the male sling. In fact, Kumar et al. reported that when men with post-prostatectomy incontinence were offered a choice of AUS and male sling, 92 % of patients chose the sling in order to avoid using a mechanical device [20].

Manual dexterity and patient understanding should be assessed prior to surgical intervention. Adequate use of an AUS requires regular and reliable fine motor skills to manipulate the pump, which is typically located in the dependent portion of the scrotum. While the exact cutoff for the minimum dexterity needed is nebulous, one should exercise caution if considering AUS placement in patients with advanced age or a progressive neurological disease. Although caretakers can manage the artificial urinary sphincter if necessary, relying on others in these situations is generally precarious. As patients age, the device can be deactivated if the patient cannot manage the pump, but this would lead to recurrent incontinence. As the age of the population continues to rise, additional patients and their caregivers will likely be faced with these situations. While further study is needed to ascertain the safest course, communication between patient and family members is key while patients are independent and active. This may help prevent, for example, inadvertent catheterization with an activated AUS leading to increased morbidity for patients unable to fully participate in their own healthcare related decisions. Advising patients to consider the benefits of a medical ID bracelet may mitigate some of these issues.

A general medical history should also be elicited from the patient. Given the consequences of infection, patients at higher risk such as those with diabetics or who are immunocompromised should be identified and counseled carefully.Hyperglycemia in the perioperative period for various surgeries has been associated with longer hospital stay, higher health care resource utilization and greater perioperative mortality [21]. It remains controversial if tight glycemic control in the perioperative and postoperative period is beneficial, but certainly conventional glycemic control is generally considered the current standard [22]. Those patients with a history of prior implant infection, evidence of frequent unexplained infections or an immunocompromised state may benefit from infectious disease consult prior to consideration of AUS implantation. Patients with rheumatoid arthritis or inflammatory bowel disease on immunomodulators may consider a drug holiday in partnership with their prescribing physician. In summary, these special populations should be appropriately counseled regarding the potential increased morbidity and mortality associated with implantation surgery.

Erectile dysfunction, which is relatively more common than incontinence after prostatectomy, should be evaluated during the clinic visit. While there are numerous medical therapies for ED, if it remains refractory, the most definitive surgical treatment is penile prosthesis. While some surgeons have reservations regarding simultaneous AUS and penile prosthesis placement given possible increased risk of infection, multiple studies have demonstrated that it is safe with similar perioperative and subjective outcomes [23, 24].

Performing an appropriate physical exam is an important step before incontinence surgery. While likely identified during thorough history taking, it is important to note any prior surgical incisions or abnormal anatomy, which can be critical for operative planning. For example, noting that a minimally invasive (typically transperitoneal) or open (typically extraperitoneal) approach had been undertaken for previous radical prostatectomy may help the surgeon in determining reservoir placement. Additionally, the patient should be checked for an inguinal hernia, which may require repair or change the expected location of the reservoir. Alternative causes of incontinence can be evaluated or ruled out by testing for perineal sensation, bulbocavernosus reflex or rectal exam. Additionally, it is important to examine the operative area to ensure there are no active skin infections or anatomic abnormalities that would preclude surgery. An informal assessment of a patient's digital manipulation skills can usually be performed passively during an encounter, but if any tremor or weakness is suspected, a full neurologic exam or referral would be appropriate. In a female, a thorough pelvic exam is necessary to evaluate for Valsalva-induced leakage before undergoing any surgical interventions for stress incontinence.

Preoperative Testing

An incontinence evaluation generally includes urine studies, a voiding diary and may also include an assessment of post-void residual. Cystoscopy is often performed prior to surgery to delineate anatomy and rule out stricture disease. Post-prostatectomy patients with incontinence should be evaluated for bladder neck contracture. Studies have estimated the incidence of bladder neck contracture at 1.1–1.4 % after robotic prostatectomy [25, 26], which seems to be slightly lower than the reported rates of 2.5–2.6 % for open retropubic prostatectomy [26, 27]. Any stricture or bladder neck contracture should be treated and monitored for recurrence prior to surgery. AUS in patients with history of prior urethral stricture should be performed with great caution as endoscopic treatments, such as urethrotomy for simple urethral strictures, are associated with a high recurrence rate with a median time to recurrence of 9 months [28].

Prior to AUS placement, a few basic laboratory studies should be performed. A basic metabolic panel and complete blood count assess for renal function, leukocytosis, and thrombocytopenia. If diabetic, a hemoglobin A1C can assist in ascertaining the patient's 3-month glucose control. Poorly controlled diabetics are at a greater risk for infectious complications. In addition, routine urinalysis and/or culture should be performed to rule out infection or bacteriuria, both of which should be treated prior to surgery.

Urodynamic studies (UDS) prior to AUS placement are a matter of some debate. Certainly if needed to confirm the diagnosis or rule out alternative etiologies, UDS can be of considerable utility. In the setting of post-prostatectomy incontinence, preoperative urodynamics is generally left to surgeon preference. While detrusor underactivity is relatively common after radical prostatectomy [29], multiple studies have demonstrated that adverse preoperative urodynamic features do not negatively affect continence results after AUS placement [30, 31]. If not undergoing preoperative cystoscopy, urodynamics can add useful anatomic information. For example, in a study of 169 men with post-prostatectomy incontinence, 32 men (19 %) did not have demonstrable incontinence while the UDS catheter was in place but had leakage after the catheter was removed. Of these 32 patients, 18 men (56 %) were found to have an anastomotic stricture [32].

Considerations with Prior Incontinence Surgery

For patients with prior incontinence surgery, surgeons should pursue a thorough preoperative workup. Similar to the workup for a patient without prior incontinence surgery, ascertaining the degree of leakage is key. A complete history regarding timing and duration of failure may hint at the etiology. For example, the patient may simply not be operating the AUS correctly so the exact technique should be demonstrated by the patient and observed by the physician. Cystoscopy is mandatory in the setting of a prior AUS to evaluate for erosion, mechanical failure, stricture and urethral atrophy. While visualizing the area of the artificial sphincter, the device should be cycled. If the device is confirmed to be working appropriately, then alternative diagnoses should be entertained. Urethral atrophy can be identified in this manner. If the device does not cycle, a leak of filling solution may have occurred. This can be determined by performing an abdominal ultrasound or if a filling solution of diluted contrast was used during the initial procedure, an abdominal X-ray can identify an appropriately filled reservoir. In the setting of a functional, appropriately managed AUS, urodynamic studies may reveal adverse findings such as detrusor overactivity or poor compliance, which may identify a treatable etiology and prevent unnecessary surgical intervention.

Urethral atrophy is a common cause of recurrent incontinence after AUS. There is some controversy regarding the optimal management. The options include cuff downsizing [33], relocation of the cuff proximally [34], transcorporal placement [35], or use of a tandem cuff [36]. Comparative studies are unfortunately lacking. Therefore, ultimately, treatment is decided based on anatomic considerations and surgeon preference. Regardless, large series have shown favorable results for secondary sphincter implantation compared to primary AUS placement [37].

It is important to remember that recurrent incontinence due to mechanical malfunction of an indwelling artificial urinary sphincter does not obligate surgical intervention. If no erosion or infection is discovered, it is ultimately a decision made between the patient and surgeon. If improving the patient's incontinence, likely in the form of complete device replacement, is worth the known risks and complications then reoperation should occur. At the very least, device malfunction is not an emergency and careful decision making and operative planning can commence prior to surgical revision.

Practice Models, Patterns and Learning Curve

The management of patients with post-prostatectomy incontinence remains non-standardized, and male incontinence surgery is generally underutilized. This may be secondary to feelings of embarrassment, belief that treatment is futile or lack of knowledge regarding management options. Reynolds et al. demonstrated considerable state and regional variation in the use of AUS even when controlling for differences in rates of prostatectomy and distribution of urologists, suggesting underutilization in certain areas of the country [38]. Similarly, considerable variation in the performance of AUS has been demonstrated on an international level [39]. Even though the overall number of incontinence procedures has steadily risen with time [40], only a small minority of surgeons perform a high volume of artificial urinary sphincter cases. Additionally, Kim et al. reported that in a population based cohort of older men, only 6 % of men underwent an incontinence procedure after prostatectomy [41]. Multiple issues may be playing a role. In addition to patient factors such as patient perception or misconception, surgeon availability, and expertise to perform the procedure may also limit AUS placement in otherwise viable operative candidates.

The learning curve for the placement of artificial urinary sphincter remains controversial. While one single surgeon study suggested a learning curve of AUS was roughly 25 cases [42], a larger study with multiple surgeons demonstrated a slow but steady decrease in reoperative rates showing no plateau through 200 procedures, indicating a prolonged learning curve [43]. The majority of patients were treated by surgeons who had performed a total of ≤25 AUS placements with only 9 % seeing a surgeon with ≥100 prior procedures [43]. Similarly, Lee et al. reported that over 90 % of AUS cases are done by surgeons who performed five or fewer each year [44]. As a result, there may be considerable room for preventable cases of reoperation for this reconstructive surgery. One study demonstrated the feasibility of a formal regional referral service for post-prostatectomy incontinence, which can lead to standardized, high level care from specialized urologic centers [45].

Surgical Technique

Preparation

Various steps should be taken prior to artificial urinary sphincter insertion. While ruling out urinary or cutaneous infections is imperative before incontinence surgery, many surgeons choose to prescribe a topical home antimicrobial regimen before the patients arrive in the hospital. In fact, employing a chlorhexidine based 5-day preoperative scrub has been shown to decrease bacterial skin colonization compared to traditional soap and water for patients undergoing AUS insertion [46].

On the day of surgery, hair removal is necessary prior to skin cleaning and incision. A Cochrane review regarding preoperative hair removal concluded that clippers were associated with fewer surgical site infections than shaving with a razor [47]. These recommendations should be followed on the day of surgery to minimize infectious risks.

Intravenous prophylactic antibiotics should be given prior to skin incision. Various recommendations (such as vancomycin with gentamicin or cephalosporin with gentamicin) have been published regarding ideal antibiotic choice prior to genitourinary prosthetic surgery [48]. The regimen should generally garner broad antimicrobial coverage against skin and urinary organisms and can

be modified in regard to local resistance patterns and patient allergies. Intravenous antibiotics are generally continued for 24 h, and many surgeons choose to keep patients on some oral antimicrobial for up to 1 week after discharge. Extended duration prophylaxis (>24 h) in this setting has not been well studied and should be approached with some caution given the theoretical, though admittedly low, risks of adverse events such as resistant bacteria or *Clostridium difficile* colitis. As mentioned previously, special populations, such as patients with history of previous prosthetic infections, patients who are immunocompromised or those on immunomodulating drugs, may benefit from infectious disease consultation to assist in antibiotic selection and duration.

Preoperative antimicrobial topical surgical site preparation is critical in establishing a sterile operative field. While choice of cleansing solution varies in surgical practice, a randomized controlled trial has shown chlorhexidine–alcohol to be superior to povidone–iodine in terms of superficial and deep incisional infections for clean-contaminated cases [49]. Specifically for genitourinary prosthetic surgery, chlorhexidine–alcohol has also been shown to be superior to povidone–iodine in terms of eliminating skin flora based on preoperative and postoperative cultures [50]. Some authors recommend an extended time for surgical scrubbing (10–15 min). Though this has not been well studied, there would seem to be little downside other than the few additional minutes of anesthesia.

AUS in the Bulbar Urethra

If not performed preoperatively, cystoscopy may be performed at the start of the procedure to rule out stricture disease. A 14 French Foley catheter is inserted on the sterile field, which facilitates identification and dissection of the urethra as well as possibly providing standardized sizing while choosing the appropriately sized cuff. The bladder should be drained for reservoir placement. Although urine is theoretically sterile, urine contamination into the operative field can be limited by utilizing gravity bag drainage as opposed to the suction tip, which will be used later in the operative field.

Incision and Urethral Dissection

The usual location of the incision is the perineum just inferior to the scrotum. A midline, longitudinal incision is made over the urethra, which can be palpated with the urethral catheter in place. The incision is extended 4–6 cm but should not approach the anus, which is ubiquitously colonized with bacteria and should be excluded by the surgical drapes. A marking skin staple can be used to ensure the surgeon is aware of the most caudal extent of the operative field. A Turner-Warwick retractor can be used to optimize exposure of relevant anatomy. Electrocautery is used to minimize bleeding in the operative field until the bulbospongiosus is encountered. The surgeon should switch to sharp dissection with Metzenbaum scissors to divide the bulbospongiosus to visualize the urethra. Great care should be taken during urethral dissection. Generally, blunt dissection or "spreading" should be avoided when mobilizing the dorsal aspect of the urethra. Instead, controlled sharp dissection using Metzenbaum scissors, with the urethra under lateral tension, is preferred to minimize the risk of urethral laceration.

The location of the cuff has been historically in one of two positions. For post-prostatectomy patients, the location is typically the bulbar urethra (Fig. 5.2). Surgical dissection for bulbar urethral placement is relatively straightforward using the perineal approach. However, an upper transverse transscrotal approach remains an alternative with the advantage of placing the reservoir through the same incision [51]. There is some evidence that the perineal approach provides superior outcomes compared to a transscrotal approach [52]. The bladder neck is the alternative location, which is typically used in women and children, and is also often preferred in men with an intact prostate (Fig. 5.3). Of note, a bladder neck cuff is contraindicated for post prostatectomy incontinence. For men, it is generally reserved for patients with neurologic etiologies

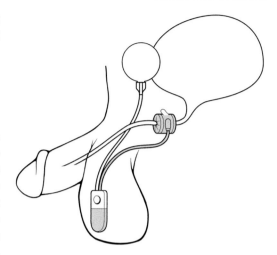

Fig. 5.2 Bulbar urethra placement of the AUS (courtesy of AMS)

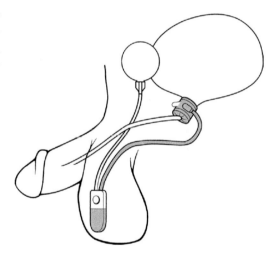

Fig. 5.3 Bladder neck placement of AUS (courtesy of AMS)

of incontinence such as neurogenic bladder or exstrophy. Dissection of the urethra is more challenging for bladder neck placement as it requires circumferential dissection of the urethra at the junction of the bladder and prostate. If bladder neck placement is desired for the cuff, a variety of alternative surgical approaches may be pursued. For example, studies have shown satisfactory results with a number of approaches including abdominal [53], vaginal [54], purely laparoscopic [55], and robotic techniques in both men [56] and women [57, 58].

Device Preparation

Careful technique should be used during preparation of the various system components of the AUS. This ensures that free air is not introduced into the system, which can cause malfunction due to lockout. The first step involves preparation of the control pump. The two ends of the control pump tubing are placing in a basin with filling solution. The pump is repeatedly squeezed while keeping the tips of the tubing submerged and the tubing of the control pump in a 45° angle upwards. After all internal air in the pump and tubing has been expelled, tubing-shod mosquito hemostats should be applied a few centimeters from each end. Of note, only one ratchet click on each hemostat should be applied to maintain occlusive pressure without providing excessive force, which can damage the tubing. For antibiotic coated devices, the pump should be placed away from any other instruments and covered with a sterile drape until implantation.

The pressure regulating balloon should be prepared next. The balloon should be deflated manually. A 15 gauge blunt tip needle attached to a 30 mL syringe filled while 25 mL of fluid is inserted into the tubing then withdrawn to completely deflate the balloon. The balloon is then inflated with 20 mL of fluid. The balloon is rotated and the fluid and any air should be withdrawn to remove all possible air. A tubing-shod hemostat is then placed on the tubing again with only one click.

The cuff is the prepared in a similar fashion by attaching a blunt tipped 30 mL syringe, this time with 10 mL of fluid. The cuff should be completely deflated manually by withdrawing the syringe, then 3–4 mL of fluid (depending on the cuff size) should be instilled. Air bubbles should be manipulated manually out of the cuff while holding the syringe and tubing upright to allow them to escape into the superior aspect of the syringe. This can be repeated although overfilling the cuff should be avoided. After all air has been removed, apply two tubing-shod hemostats a few centimeters away from each other a few centimeters from the end of the tubing. The cuff should also then be set-aside in a dry, safe place under a sterile drape.

While device preparation is sometimes relegated to the surgical scrub nurse or other non-urologic personnel, it remains a critical step in urologic prosthetic surgery placement, and improper technique can lead to device malfunction or infection. This is especially true for smaller volume hospitals with rotating surgical teams, where an inexperienced individual may be the scrubbed assistant. Dedicated urologic nursing or ownership of the preparation portion of the procedure by the urologist can mitigate this effect. Critical steps include proper technique during removal of air bubbles from the multiple components of the device, which can prevent air locks and malfunctions. Generalized handling of the device is also extremely important to minimize complications. This includes appropriate clamping in terms of equipment (tubing-shod mosquito hemostats), positioning of the mosquito hemostats and use of a single ratchet click. Additionally, the device should be prepared and stored away from the rest of the operative tray, which may include sharp instruments that could damage the device. Finally, minimizing handling may limit the risk of inadvertent contamination, and this may be a strong argument towards having just one experienced urologist prepare and implant the device itself.

The AMS 800 can be filled with normal saline or radiographically opaque contrast. It is critical that if using contrast, sterile water (not saline) should be added in a specific amount to achieve an isotonic solution. Table 5.1 specifies the exact amount of contrast media and sterile water to mix. For example, when using Conray 43 (Mallinckrodt, Dublin, Ireland), 30 cc of contrast should be used with 60 cc of sterile H_2O to create an appropriate dilution. The use of contrast in this setting is contraindicated in patients with iodine allergy.

Cuff Sizing and Placement

After urethral dissection, the circumference of the urethra is measuring using the provided cuff sizer. Sizing should be performed around the corpus spongiosum with or without the catheter in

Table 5.1 Recommended dilutions if using contrast for AUS filling (courtesy of AMS)

Contrast media	Dilution			Manufacturer	Validated for InhibiZone use
Conray 43	30 cc Conray 43	+	60 cc sterile H_2O	Mallinckrodt	Yes
Cysto Conray II	60 cc Cysto Conray II	+	15 cc sterile H_2O	Mallinckrodt	Yes
Hypaque-Cysto	60 cc Hypaque-Cysto	+	58 cc sterile H_2O	Nycomed	No
Isovue 200	60 cc Isovue 200	+	23 cc sterile H_2O	Bracco	No
Isovue 300	57 cc Isovue 300	+	60 cc sterile H_2O	Bracco	No
Isovue 370	38 cc Isovue 370	+	60 cc sterile H_2O	Bracco	No
Omnipaque 180	60 cc Omnipaque 180	+	14 cc sterile H_2O	Nycomed	No
Omnipaque 240	60 cc Omnipaque 240	+	38 cc sterile H_2O	Nycomed	No
Omnipaque 300	57 cc Omnipaque 300	+	60 cc sterile H_2O	Nycomed	Yes
Omnipaque 350	48 cc Omnipaque 350	+	60 cc sterile H_2O	Nycomed	No
Telebrix 12	53 cc Telebrix 12	+	47 cc sterile H_2O	Laboratoire Guerbel	Yes

place. While this is generally surgeon preference, one method should be used to maintain consistency of measurements for a single surgeon. Of note, the circumference of the inside of the sizer is slightly smaller than the outer circumference.

Determining the correct size of the cuff is critical to ensure appropriate coaptation of the urethra when the device is activated. Sizes vary from 3.5 to 11.0 cm in circumference. The 3.5 cm cuff has only been available since late 2009. The larger sizes are generally reserved for bladder neck placement. While many urologists favor implanting a cuff of the exact size that is measured, it is sometimes necessary or appropriate to choose a size slightly larger. One advantage of a larger size is to mitigate the risk of postoperative urinary retention, minimize the development of urethral atrophy or prevent risk of future erosion. The concern of placing a cuff too large is leaving the patient with ineffective urethral coaptation and poor continence results. However, there is some evidence that modest upsizing results in similar short-term continence and satisfaction while improving long term outcomes [59]. In the setting of urethral atrophy, a relatively standard 4.0–4.5 cm cuff may appear to be too large. Alternative operative techniques to deal with this clinical situation include placing a tandem cuff [36], urethral buttressing [60], or transcorporal placement [35]. Transcorporal placement involves additional dissection and will be discussed later. Especially in those patients with previous radiation, caution should be exercised

when using a very tight cuff as radiation has been shown to significantly increase the risk of erosion when using the 3.5 cm cuff compared to larger sizes [61].

Once the desired size is determined, the cuff should be passed tab first under the urethra and the tubing should be passed through the tab hole to completely surround the urethra. Multiple shod hemostats are needed to successfully wrap the cuff around the urethra. Finally, the tab should be pulled over the tubing adapter (which appears as a button), which locks the cuff in position. Failure to adequately fasten the cuff can ultimately lead to failure if the cuff becomes unfastened. The small bit of tail remaining after fastening can be excised with blunt tipped scissors or left in place based on surgeon preference.

Reservoir Placement

Multiple alternative methods have been described for placement of the pressure regulating balloon such as scrotal or perineal, but a separate abdominal incision is generally recommended. After skin incision, Army Navy retractors are used to sweep away the superficial layers to reveal the anterior rectus or external oblique fascia. This is incised to allow separation of the muscle. Blunt finger dissection is usually sufficient to create adequate space in the space of Retzius for the balloon. When possible, preplacing fascial sutures prior to introducing the device can avoid inadvertent puncture. For prosthetic cases, absorbable monofilament suture may help to minimize infectious risks. When closing fascia, polydioxanone (PDS) suture is ideal given its longer time for absorption. For superficial layers including skin, faster absorbing suture is recommended.

A 61–70 cm H_2O pressure regulating balloon is generally recommended for bulbar urethral cuff placement with 71–80 cm H_2O reserved for cuffs at the bladder neck, which require a higher pressure to maintain closure. A deflated reservoir is inserted through the fascial defect, and the sutures are then tied around the tubing. Regardless of using normal saline or a diluted contrast, 22–24 mL of fluid is generally used to fill the pressure regulating balloon.

Pump Placement

Attention should next be turned to placement of the manual control pump. Through the incision for reservoir placement, blunt dissection is carried inferiorly into a dependent portion of the ipsilateral portion of the scrotum. It is important to avoid a superficial dissection (above Scarpa's fascia), which can lead to palpable components and increase the risk of erosion. Great care should also be taken to avoid the testicular vessels. After the subdartos pouch is created, the pump is lowered into the space with the tubing visible from the incision. Figure 5.4 demonstrates this dissection.

Connections

Connections are generally made through the abdominal incision. This includes connecting the tubing from the cuff to the pump (translucent clear) as well as the reservoir to the pump (clear with black stripes). The connections must be made carefully to avoid any pitfalls that could result in mechanical dysfunction. The AMS Quick Connect Sutureless Window Connectors have replaced the previous suture-tie connectors, which can still be used if necessary. The various shapes of connectors are

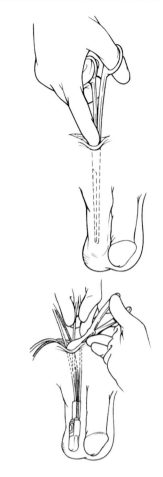

Fig. 5.4 Dissection for control pump (courtesy of AMS)

shown in Fig. 5.5. The tubing should be cut using a straight scissors transversely to create a flat surface. It is important to instill saline into the components of the connector to avoid any air bubbles from being trapped internally. Additionally, multiple tubing-shod mosquito hemostats should be kept a few centimeters from the end of the tubing until the connection is completed. The collet rings are slipped over each end of the tubing with the teeth toward the middle, and the tubing is then inserted as far as possible until the central stop of the middle connector (Fig. 5.6). Through the two small windows, the tubing should be visible. At this point, the two collet rings should be seated into the middle connector and the squeeze tool should be applied in a fashion as to not trap any tubing material in the jaws. The squeeze tool is closed

Fig. 5.5 Various quick connectors for AUS placement (courtesy of AMS)

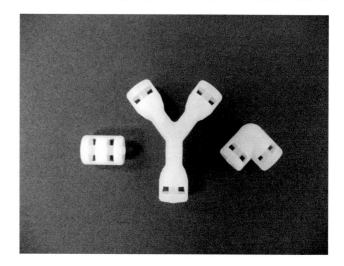

Fig. 5.6 Proper technique for insertion of tubing (courtesy of AMS)

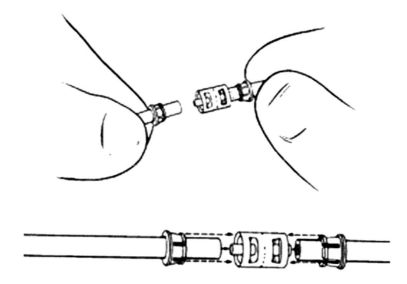

until the closure stops are flush with the central connector (Fig. 5.7). If using a straight connector, this is one application of the tool, but for right angle connections, the tool must be used twice (once for each side). After all the connections are complete, the hemostats should be removed, and the device should be tested for appropriate cycling.

Closure and Follow-Up

At the end of the procedure, the device should be left in a deactivated state with the cuff deflated. All incisions should be irrigated and closed with absorbable monofilament suture to minimize infectious risks. A multilayer closure can theoretically protect patients with superficial skin infections from deep prosthetic infections, and skin glue creates a watertight barrier for incisions.

While some surgeons do treat younger, healthier patients as outpatients, others utilize an overnight stay as a routine. An inpatient stay allows for management/monitoring of comorbidities, more rigorous assessment of adequate voiding prior to discharge, longer course of intravenous antibiotics and intravenous pain medication if needed. For outpatients, the patient should be left without a catheter, and the patient should demonstrate

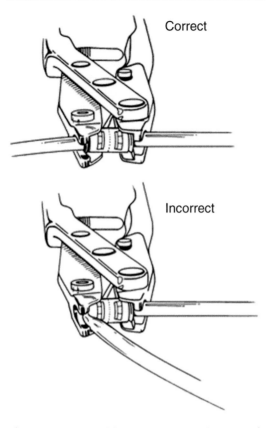

Correct

Incorrect

Fig. 5.7 Squeeze tool for quick connectors (courtesy of AMS)

adequate voiding prior to discharge. Some surgeons insist on a documented post-void residual while others assess this clinically. For an overnight hospital stay, some surgeons prefer to leave the patient with a small (usually 12–14 Fr) indwelling urethral catheter and then perform a voiding trial in the morning. Others allow immediate voiding after surgery.

Once the patient has demonstrated adequate voiding and pain control, the patient should be discharged. Some endorse an initial regimen of pulling the pump inferiorly in the scrotum every few days to minimize upward migration into the inguinal canal. The downside of this approach includes additional pain related to manipulation as well as inadvertent activation of the device.

The length of antibiotics after surgery remains an area of debate. Many surgeons prefer to send patients home on a week of an antibiotic with urinary and skin coverage. However, prolonged (>24 h) antimicrobial prophylaxis for AUS should be approached with some caution as no studies have proven their effectiveness in the face of theoretical risks.

The cuff should remain deactivated and the patient generally returns for device activation in 4–6 weeks after surgery. This time frame allows for adequate initial healing of the urethra to avoid erosion as well as the time necessary to avoid pain with pump manipulation. The patient can rely on absorbent pads or condom catheter during this time and should notify their surgeon if any fevers, inordinate bruising, purulent drainage, or skin infections occur after surgery.

Long-term management requires diligence from the patient. Patients should not be catheterized without device deactivation or a significant risk of urethral erosion exists, which usually requires device explantation if erosion occurs. This should be stressed repeatedly with the patient and any associated caregivers. Some patients wear an identification band indicating the presence of an AUS. However, inevitably, patients in critical condition with an AUS occasionally undergo attempted urethral catheter placement by an unknowing provider. Such attempts with the device still activated are usually met with some tactile resistance at the level of the cuff. This is therefore sometimes discovered at the time of catheter placement if the catheter will not pass, but AUS problems can also be noted after catheter removal in relation to subsequent erosion or infectious sequelae.

Special Circumstances

Transcorporal Cuff

Transcorporal placement of the cuff of the AUS remains an option for difficult initial or revision surgery. It can be especially useful in the setting of prior erosion or urethral atrophy where usual cuff sizes do not allow an appropriately snug fit with the urethra. Instead of dissecting around the bulbospongiosus muscle dorsally, two longitudinal incisions are made on the tunica albuginea of the ventral surface of the corpus cavernosa. This allows the dorsal aspect of the cuff to pass through medial corporal lining of each corporal

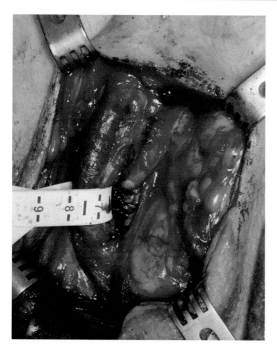

Fig. 5.8 Intraoperative dissection during transcorporal AUS placement

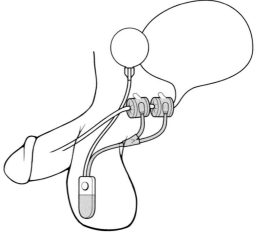

Fig. 5.9 Tandem cuff AUS (courtesy of AMS)

body as well as through the septum between the corporal cylinders. The lateral edges of the corporotomies require sutures, which should be pre-placed, to assist in retraction and eventually to close the corporal defects [35]. A representative dissection for transcorporal AUS placement is shown in Fig. 5.8. In general, transcorporal placement should only be performed for impotent men given the potential risk of postoperative erectile dysfunction associated with the dissection.

Tandem Cuff

While the usual AUS placement entails a single occlusive inflatable cuff, utilizing a double (or tandem) urethral cuff is an option. The exact role and benefit of tandem cuffs remains controversial among reconstructive urologists. This is largely due to a relative lack of comparative studies, especially in a prospective manner. In theory, a tandem cuff creates two levels of (and perhaps greater) occlusive forces, which could improve continence outcomes. However, given two separate cuffs interacting with the urethra, one downside is an additional risk of erosion or infection.

Two areas of dissection are required, with the additional site typically 1 cm distal to the usual location at the bulbar urethral sphincter (Fig. 5.9). It is possible to perform the second dissection more proximally if the initial dissection was somewhat distal and the patient has adequate urethral length. A 1 cm distance between cuffs is usually recommended to avoid interaction between the cuffs and tissue ischemia in the intervening urethra. To place a tandem cuff, a Y-connector is used with the long portion facing the control pump. Additional solution is required for filling if tandem cuff placement is being performed, and 24–26 mL is generally recommended for the pressure regulating balloon.

There is some controversy about the benefit of double cuff placement. However, while feasibility has been shown in many studies, long term studies have shown no difference in clinical outcomes between initial single vs. double cuff placement in post-prostatectomy patients with some concern of higher complication rates when using two cuffs [62].

Bladder Neck Placement

Men with intact prostates and stress incontinence as well as women with stress incontinence with intrinsic sphincter deficiency are appropriate candidates for AUS placement after failure of medical and surgical therapy [63]. Just as with the bulbar urethra, patients require the necessary sophistication and manual dexterity to use the device, proper motivation and be significantly bothered by their lack of urinary control. The procedure and outcomes for women or men with cuffs at the bladder neck differ from those in the bulbar urethra due to anatomic, physiologic, and technical concerns that deserve special consideration.

The technique for AMS 800 implantation at the bladder neck requires a different approach for accessing the urethra. One approach involves a transverse abdominal incision with dissection of the space of Retzius and exposure of the endopelvic fascia. The bladder neck is then dissected at the level of the catheter balloon for circumferential dissection of the proximal urethra. Many men and women who are candidates for AUS have a history of previous failed surgery. Therefore, adhesions may be encountered during this key part of the procedure. Dense adhesions in the space of Retzius or surrounding the bladder neck increase the risk for vaginal, rectal or bladder injuries. If vesical or vaginal injuries are encountered some practitioners choose to close these primarily and continue while others choose procedure abandonment because of higher erosion rates with such injuries [64]. Bladder neck implantation commonly requires larger cuffs ($\geq$5 cm). For women, a space is developed in the labia majora, and the pump may be placed in this location. For men, the pump is placed in the inferior aspect of the scrotum, similar to previously described. The reservoir is placed in a lateral vesicle space. A similar approach using minimally invasive laparoscopic techniques such as laparoscopy or robotics has also been successful [55, 57]. Moreover, some choose to approach the bladder neck in women transvaginally [54]. Except for the anatomic details above, device preparation itself is generally similar regardless of location of the cuff.

Operative Considerations

Revision Surgery

When operating with an artificial urinary sphincter already in place, the surgical approach is slightly different. A pseudocapsule surrounds the various components, which can actually make dissection easier. Given the various reasons to perform reoperative surgery, gross infection is one of the most challenging. When gross infection necessitates device explantation, purulent fluid and debris is often encountered, and the patient should undergo removal of all components and a thorough antibiotic washout.

In the setting of an AUS revision, the majority of procedures involve complete removal and replacement of the entire device. This is especially true if more than 1–2 years have elapsed from the initial surgery. As the device has an unavoidable mechanical failure rate that increases over time, revision represents an opportunity to postpone a future procedure for device failure of a currently functioning component. Resetting the clock on a patient's entire AUS by completely replacing all the components is thereby generally recommended. Additionally, the AMS Quick Connect Sutureless Window Connectors are not designed to be used for revision surgeries where the entire device is not replaced given the changes in tubing integrity over time. In these situations, a sutured approach may be utilized. Finally, while uncommon, simply finding one correctable problem with a patient's AUS does not preclude an issue with two different components, and both of these issues would be addressed by replacing the entire device.

Occasionally, in the setting of either prosthetic replacement or subtotal device removal for noninfectious reasons, the dissection of the pressure regulating balloon proves exceedingly challenging. In an effort to avoid an abdominal counterincision, injury to the bladder, or inadvertent damage to vascular structures, some surgeons may opt to drain the reservoir, cut the tubing as proximally as possible and leave the defunctionalized pressure regulating balloon in place. While there may be theoretical risks of infectious complications or untoward events related to device migration, two prior series have demonstrated that intentionally leaving a reservoir is generally safe [65, 66]. However, the authors of this chapter generally advise against leaving defunctionalized components in patients when removal is safe and feasible.

Urethral Injury

Urethral injury is a risk during dissection of the space needed for the inflatable cuff. This can often occur dorsally if choosing to perform blind blunt dissection of the urethra. Recognition of the injury, which can be performed by visualizing the catheter or by pericatheter instillation of fluid or methylene blue, is critical. Injuring the urethra is generally recognized as a contraindication to continuing AUS placement and the procedure should be aborted. Proceeding with immediate AUS placement is associated with considerable risk of urethral erosion, especially if the cuff is placed at the site of injury. The injury should be repaired using absorbable suture and a catheter left in place for healing. AUS placement can be attempted again after confirming an appropriately healed urethra.

Rectal Injury

Visualizing and injuring the rectum during urethral dissection is more common for bladder neck placement given the difficult dissection needed at the vesicourethral junction. Rectal injury during AUS placement is considered an absolute contraindication to proceeding with prosthetic placement given the considerable associated infectious risks. The rectum should be repaired with general surgery consultation if necessary, and AUS placement should only be attempted again months later after confirming complete healing. In the setting of uncomplicated AUS placement for patients with prior posterior distraction injuries, subsequent erosion into the rectum has been reported [67].

Perioperative Complications and Management

Urinary Retention

Immediate postoperative urinary retention is an infrequent complication after artificial urinary sphincter placement and may occur even though the cuff is deactivated after placement. While the etiology of retention is often unknown, edema or hematoma around the cuff may be a contributing cause. The risk of postoperative urinary retention for ≥4 cm cuffs has been reported at 8 % with the rate of retention can be as high as 32 % for transcorporal placement [68]. Management includes first ensuring that the cuff is deactivated. Initially, some surgeons choose to perform gentle clean intermittent catheterization to allow for a repeat voiding trial while others place a urethral catheter for a short period of time (<24 h). Regardless, prolonged inability to void should be managed with suprapubic tube placement to prevent the risk of urethral erosion due to catheterization while the swelling subsides. Though not specific to the immediate postoperative period, Seideman et al. demonstrated that prolonged urinary catheterization (mostly commonly for nongenitourinary surgery or retention) was an independent risk factor for AUS cuff erosion [69]. Suprapubic tube placement can be performed using cystoscopic and/or ultrasound guidance, but an open approach may be safer to avoid inadvertent damage to any AUS components. Smith et al. reported the need of suprapubic tube in only 1 of 53 patients treated with a ≥4 cm cuff [68].

Infection

Infection of the AUS can result from bacterial seeding at the time of implantation, hematogenous spread from septic events or from erosion into a non-sterile space. Mostly commonly, bacteria involved originate from the skin or urethral contents. Contemporary series have shown that Staphylococcus aureus is the most commonly cultured bacteria with a considerable amount of methicillin resistance observed [70]. The standard of care with any deep or prosthetic infection is surgical removal of all prosthetic components and antibiotic administration. For very minor superficial skin infections immediately after placement of an AUS, an attempt at treatment with antibiotics can be made with close monitoring if a multilayer closure was performed, but any progression of infection should be managed aggressively with explantation.

Immediate Mechanical Failure

Immediate mechanical device malfunction is a relatively uncommon problem after artificial urinary sphincter placement. In general, it can result from incorrect surgical technique. Some of the etiologies include inadvertent puncture of the device during the procedure, unsuccessful connection of the various components of the device or inappropriate filling of the reservoir. This complication is generally discovered after initial device activation at 4–6 weeks and is confirmed by visualizing absent cuff coaptation on urethroscopy. The device should be revised when mechanical failures have occurred as these issues will not repair themselves.

Long-Term Complications

Mechanical Failure

As the AUS is a mechanical device, it is subject to mechanical malfunction over time. This can result from breakage of the lining of one or more of the components, tubing breakdown, any other cause of fluid loss or an issue with the valve mechanism of the control pump. Estimates of the rates of mechanical failure range from 7.6 to 21 % in long-term studies [71, 72]. Advances in design (such as the narrow backed cuff) have decreased the failure rates over time. The rate of mechanical malfunction generally increases with the length of time since initial implantation.

Urethral Atrophy

One of the most common reasons for recurrent incontinence after an initially successful AUS placement is urethral atrophy. Chronic compression causes the corpus spongiosum of the urethra to become attenuated, and consequently the cuff will no longer occlude the flow of urine. The rate of urethral atrophy has been estimated at 9.6–11.4 % in long-term studies [37, 73]. The timing of recurrent incontinence can suggest a diagnosis of atrophy (median 29.6 months), which tends to

occur sooner after initial implantation when compared to mechanical failure (median 68.1 months) [73]. The diagnosis is typically made during evaluation for recurrent incontinence by cystoscopically visualizing the urethra and observing a lack of coaptation. The options for management include cuff downsizing, replacing the cuff in a new location, placing a tandem cuff, transcorporal placement or buttressing.

Urethral Erosion

If the urethral becomes extremely atrophic and thin, there is a risk of spontaneous urethral erosion. Additionally, in the setting of a traumatic catheterization, with or without an activated cuff, a urethral injury may occur and expose the artificial urinary sphincter to the lumen of the urethra. In this setting, patients may present with hematuria, recurrent incontinence or signs of an infection. Urethroscopy should be performed to evaluate the urethra and confirm the diagnosis. The standard of care for urethral erosion is immediate explantation of the entire device. If feasible, the site of urethral erosion should be repaired primarily at the time of device removal as Rozanski et al. have shown a benefit in terms of minimizing urethral strictures using this approach when compared to those treated with Foley catheter alone (38 % vs. 85 %) [74].

Outcomes

Bulbar Urethra

Overall, the AUS has been lauded as a success in the treatment of male stress urinary incontinence. While most patients experience improvement in leakage, a significant number of men will require additional surgical procedures for a variety of issues including recurrent incontinence, infection or erosion. Long-term studies of AUS have shown excellent functional outcomes as the majority (59–92 %) of patients had good urinary outcomes at follow-up of 6.8–10 years [75–77]. The success rate is somewhat dependent on the definition of continence employed.

Stricter definitions of urinary control result in lower reported success rates. Some authors have noted that outcomes in males undergoing primary incontinence surgery are better with the cuff at the bladder neck [77].

Patients have been queried for subjective and quality of life measures after AUS implantation. Pad use after AUS is in many ways most useful for ascertaining success of urinary outcomes for patients because it offers a point of direct comparison to preoperative functioning. For example, out of 71 patients at a mean follow-up of 7.7 years, 19 (27 %) patients used 0 pads, 23 (32 %) used 1, 11 (15 %) used 1–3, and 18 (25 %) used greater than 3 pads daily. The degree of patient satisfaction correlated with the number of pads used. In an additional study, 47 patients who underwent AUS for post-prostatectomy incontinence answered a questionnaire at a median follow-up of 6.8 years. In this report, 27 % of men reported no pad use, and 52 % reported using one pad daily [75]. In addition, the underreported phenomenon of urinary leakage during sexual activity often affects men after prostatectomy. In a novel study, small numbers of men undergoing an AUS were questioned regarding potential improvement in their sexual quality of life, with the majority indicating improvement [78].

In terms of overall complication rates, estimates of revision-free device survival for post-prostatectomy males vary between (66–83 %) at 7–10 years follow-up [75–77], but the majority of revisions are within the first 2 years [75]. Of 323 patients who received AUS at the Mayo Clinic, 234 (72 %) required no surgical intervention at a mean follow-up of 68.8 months, which highlights the fact that the majority of patients experience long-term success [72].

Linder et al. reported the outcomes of 69 AUS reimplantation procedures performed for erosion or infection compared to 497 primary AUS implantations at the Mayo Clinic [79]. With median follow-up of 34 months, patients with prior AUS explantation for erosion or infection experienced an increased rate of recurrent erosion or infection compared to primary AUS implantation (19 % vs. 6.4 %). In spite of this, the 5-year overall device survival rate was 68 % for

reimplantation, which was similar to primary implantation (76 %).

Robotic implantation of AUS is a novel technique emerging as the next frontier for AUS placement with bladder neck cuff location. Six patients with neurogenic injury from spinal cord injury underwent a transperitoneal approach for AUS placement around the bladder neck. In this limited series, with median follow-up of 13 months, no early erosion, infection or device malfunction was reported. All six patients reportedly had complete continence. The advantage of robotic placement remains uncertain, as the early robotic approach accrued a median operative time of 195 min. Further long-term studies with direct comparison with other techniques are required. Moreover, robotic techniques currently have no role in the post-prostatectomy population [56].

Radiation

While some smaller studies have conflicting results, one of the largest contemporary cohorts of irradiated patients who have undergone AUS implantation was studied by Ravier et al. Early complications, defined as occurring before the sphincter was activated, were not significantly different between the 61 who did not previously have radiation therapy vs. the 61 that did receive some form of radiation therapy [16]. More erosion complications were noted in irradiated patients than in non-irradiated patients (13.1 % vs. 4.9 %). The rate of sepsis was 9.8 % and mainly occurred in irradiated patients, with a significant difference compared with non-irradiated patients (16.3 % vs. 3.2 %). In a separate single surgeon study of 176 men who underwent AUS implantation, Simhan et al. determined that the overwhelming majority of erosions for the 3.5 cm cuff occurred in irradiated men, and radiation was the only significant risk factor identified [61]. Moreover, in a meta-analysis with 36.7 months average follow-up, 579 patients underwent AUS placement after external beam radiation and radical prostatectomy vs. 1307 after radical prostatectomy alone [80]. Revision rates were higher in those that received radiation with a risk ratio of 1.56 (95 % CI: 1.02–2.72; $p < 0.05$). The authors concluded infection and/or erosion contributed to the majority of surgical revision risk compared to urethral atrophy ($p=0.020$). Interestingly, persistent urinary incontinence after implantation was greater in those patients who received radiation therapy. As such, it is best to counsel patients of additional risks if they have a history of pelvic radiation. Radiation is thought to lead to the destruction of micro-vessels in the submucosal layers via chronic hypoperfusion leading to tissue fibrosis and atrophy [81]. While the urethra is not directly targeted in pelvic radiation, nonetheless urethral tissue may be exposed and radiotoxicity may involve the urethra and surrounding tissues [82]. Additional prospective studies evaluating the impact of radiation on AUS outcomes are needed.

Individuals with prior urethroplasty are another special population with distinct anatomic considerations. In one study, 86 patients with mixed causes of compromised urethra including prior urethroplasty were evaluated after AUS placement [83]. Patients with prior urethroplasty or artificial urinary sphincter incurred a significantly increased risk of failure. In contrast, transcorporal placement did not increase risks. It is conjectured that prior urethral mobilization potentially compromises blood supply to the urethra, which predisposes patients to failure. Considering transcorporal placement in these patients who have had prior urethroplasty may be prudent.

Bladder Neck Outcomes

Outcome data is growing, and multiple series have been published on this approach. In summary, many men and women achieve continence and have high satisfaction rates after AUS placement. However, many of these studies are single center, single surgeon reports. They are limited by varied definitions of continence making attempts to directly compare results difficult. At times, subjective data on patient satisfaction is included but often with non-validated surveys.

Chung et al. presented a series of 47 consecutive women who received an AUS for the treatment of incontinence. With a mean age of 51 years, these women represented a wide range of clinical scenarios. Thirty-five of the women previously failed

anti-incontinence surgery, representative of the usual female candidates for AUS placement. Kaplan–Meier analysis showed >80 % of AUS were functioning after 100 months. Continence rates were defined strictly as dryness without pad use. By that definition, 59 % of patients reached continence with AUS only, and 85 % when clean intermittent self-catheterization was performed. In an additional contemporary series, 215 women with ISD were treated by AUS implantation [63]. In this analysis, 158 patients (73.5 %) were continent and 170 (79 %) were satisfied.

Laparoscopic approaches have been described and continence is similar to open series (80–88 %), albeit with longer operative times and shorter follow-up [55, 64, 84]. In a recent novel robotic series of six women at mean follow-up of 14 months, five were completely dry and one had transition from 4 to 1 pads daily [57].

Morbidity

Given the increased surgical challenges associated with AUS placement at the bladder neck, it is not surprising that morbidity is increased when compared with standard bulbar urethral placement. The risks of device infection, urethral erosion, urethral atrophy and mechanical failure are shared for the bulbar urethra or bladder neck implantation techniques. For those patients seeking AUS who have already have had previous surgery to the bladder neck, implantation is fraught with difficulty. There is very limited data on AUS revision surgery at the bladder neck.

In a series of 47 women, 8 (17 %) AUS were removed due to AUS erosion or infection. There were 20 AUS revisions, 16 of which were primary AUS revisions [85]. In another series, 215 women underwent AUS placement and of those, 15.3 % required reoperative procedure at a mean of 8.5 years after initial surgery. The authors discovered that risk factors associated with AUS failure were pelvic radiotherapy, age >70 year old and a previous Burch procedure [63].

In a separate series by Costa et al. of 376 AUS implantation in 344 female patients, device longevity was estimated at a mean of 14.7 years. Specifically at 5 and 10 years, device survival was 88.6 % and 69.2 %, respectively. Multivariate analysis revealed that increasing numbers of previous incontinence surgeries and a neurologic indication were independent risk factors for increased device failure [86].

Summary

The artificial urinary sphincter remains the gold standard in the treatment of post prostatectomy incontinence. While alternatives such as bulking agents or urethral slings are available and attractive for men seeking to avoid the need to manage a mechanical device, the modest success rates of these procedures have tempered their use. As prostate cancer screening guidelines continue to be refined, the rate of prostatectomy and men with subsequent incontinence may change. However, the majority of patients with post-prostatectomy incontinence who undergo AUS placement experience improved continence and are generally satisfied with the procedure. There are known perioperative and long-term risks associated with implantation that contribute to some patients requiring revision. Surgeon experience, attention to technique and even future advances in AUS technology will continue to improve outcomes and further minimize complications. It is also important that reconstructive urologists who utilize prosthetics are knowledgeable about potential pitfalls and the management of various complications. The AUS will continue to be the mainstay of treatment for male stress incontinence for the foreseeable future.

References

1. Scott FB, Bradley WE, Timm GW. Treatment of urinary incontinence by implantable prosthetic sphincter. Urology. 1973;1:252–9.
2. Foley FEB. An artificial sphincter; a new device and operation for control of enuresis and urinary incontinence. J Urol. 1947;58:250–9.
3. Carson CC. Efficacy of antibiotic impregnation of inflatable penile prostheses in decreasing infection in original implants. J Urol. 2004;171:1611–4.
4. Wilson SK, Zumbe J, Henry GD, et al. Infection reduction using antibiotic-coated inflatable penile prosthesis. Urology. 2007;70:337–40.
5. De Cógáin MR, Elliott DS. The impact of an antibiotic coating on the artificial urinary sphincter infection rate. J Urol. 2013;190:113–7.
6. Lawson TM, Amos N, Bulgen D, et al. Minocycline-induced lupus: clinical features and response to rechallenge. Rheumatology (Oxford). 2001;40: 329–35.
7. Walsh PC, Marschke P, Ricker D, et al. Patient-reported urinary continence and sexual function after anatomic radical prostatectomy. Urology. 2000;55: 58–61.
8. Stanford JL, Feng Z, Hamilton AS, et al. Urinary and sexual function after radical prostatectomy for clinically localized prostate cancer: the Prostate Cancer Outcomes Study. JAMA. 2000;283:354–60.
9. Menon M, Shrivastava A, Kaul S, et al. Vattikuti Institute prostatectomy: contemporary technique and analysis of results. Eur Urol. 2007;51:648–57. discussion 657–658.
10. Comiter C. Surgery for postprostatectomy incontinence: which procedure for which patient? Nat Rev Urol. 2015;12:91–9.
11. Nitti VW, Mourtzinos A, Brucker BM, et al. Correlation of patient perception of pad use with objective degree of incontinence measured by pad test in men with post-prostatectomy incontinence: the SUFU Pad Test Study. J Urol. 2014;192:836–42.
12. Pepper J, Zhang A, Li R, et al. Usage and results of a mobile app for managing urinary incontinence. J Urol. 2014;193:1292–7.
13. Kim YH, Kattan MW, Boone TB. Bladder leak point pressure: the measure for sphincterotomy success in spinal cord injured patients with external detrusor-sphincter dyssynergia. J Urol. 1998;159:493–6. discussion 496–497.
14. McGuire EJ, Woodside JR, Borden TA. Upper urinary tract deterioration in patients with myelodysplasia and detrusor hypertonia: a followup study. J Urol. 1983;129:823–6.
15. Gomha MA, Boone TB. Artificial urinary sphincter for post-prostatectomy incontinence in men who had prior radiotherapy: a risk and outcome analysis. J Urol. 2002;167:591–6.
16. Ravier E, Fassi-Fehri H, Crouzet S, et al. Complications after artificial urinary sphincter implantation in patients with or without prior radiotherapy. BJU Int. 2015;115:300–7.
17. Brant WO, Erickson BA, Elliott SP, et al. Risk factors for erosion of artificial urinary sphincters: a multi-center prospective study. Urology. 2014;84:934–8.
18. Fultz NH, Herzog AR. Self-reported social and emotional impact of urinary incontinence. J Am Geriatr Soc. 2001;49:892–9.
19. Moore KN, Schieman S, Ackerman T, et al. Assessing comfort, safety, and patient satisfaction with three commonly used penile compression devices. Urology. 2004;63:150–4.
20. Kumar A, Litt ER, Ballert KN, et al. Artificial urinary sphincter versus male sling for post-prostatectomy

incontinence—what do patients choose? J Urol. 2009;181:1231–5.

21. Smiley DD, Umpierrez GE. Perioperative glucose control in the diabetic or nondiabetic patient. South Med J. 2006;99:580–9. quiz 590–591.

22. Buchleitner AM, Martínez-Alonso M, Hernández M, et al. Perioperative glycaemic control for diabetic patients undergoing surgery. Cochrane Database Syst Rev. 2012;9, CD007315.

23. Mancini JG, Kizer WS, Jones LA, et al. Patient satisfaction after dual implantation of inflatable penile and artificial urinary sphincter prostheses. Urology. 2008;71:893–6.

24. Segal RL, Cabrini MR, Harris ED, et al. Combined inflatable penile prosthesis-artificial urinary sphincter implantation: no increased risk of adverse events compared to single or staged device implantation. J Urol. 2013;190:2183–8.

25. Msezane LP, Reynolds WS, Gofrit ON, et al. Bladder neck contracture after robot-assisted laparoscopic radical prostatectomy: evaluation of incidence and risk factors and impact on urinary function. J Endourol. 2008;22:97–104.

26. Breyer BN, Davis CB, Cowan JE, et al. Incidence of bladder neck contracture after robot-assisted laparoscopic and open radical prostatectomy. BJU Int. 2010;106:1734–8.

27. Erickson BA, Meeks JJ, Roehl KA, et al. Bladder neck contracture after retropubic radical prostatectomy: incidence and risk factors from a large single-surgeon experience. BJU Int. 2009;104:1615–9.

28. Santucci R, Eisenberg L. Urethrotomy has a much lower success rate than previously reported. J Urol. 2010;183:1859–62.

29. Chung DE, Dillon B, Kurta J, et al. Detrusor underactivity is prevalent after radical prostatectomy: a urodynamic study including risk factors. Can Urol Assoc J. 2012;2012:1–5.

30. Lai HH, Hsu EI, Boone TB. Urodynamic testing in evaluation of postradical prostatectomy incontinence before artificial urinary sphincter implantation. Urology. 2009;73:1264–9.

31. Thiel DD, Young PR, Broderick GA, et al. Do clinical or urodynamic parameters predict artificial urinary sphincter outcome in post-radical prostatectomy incontinence? Urology. 2007;69:315–9.

32. Weissbart SJ, Coutinho K, Chughtai B, et al. Characteristics and outcomes of men who fail to leak on intubated urodynamics prior to artificial urinary sphincter placement. Can J Urol. 2014;21:7560–4.

33. Saffarian A, Walsh K, Walsh IK, et al. Urethral atrophy after artificial urinary sphincter placement: is cuff downsizing effective? J Urol. 2003;169:567–9.

34. Couillard DR, Vapnek JM, Stone AR. Proximal artificial sphincter cuff repositioning for urethral atrophy incontinence. Urology. 1995;45:653–6.

35. Guralnick ML, Miller E, Toh KL, et al. Transcorporal artificial urinary sphincter cuff placement in cases requiring revision for erosion and urethral atrophy. J Urol. 2002;167:2075–8. discussion 2079.

36. DiMarco DS, Elliott DS. Tandem cuff artificial urinary sphincter as a salvage procedure following failed primary sphincter placement for the treatment of post-prostatectomy incontinence. J Urol. 2003;170:1252–4.

37. Raj GV, Peterson AC, Toh KL, et al. Outcomes following revisions and secondary implantation of the artificial urinary sphincter. J Urol. 2005;173:1242–5.

38. Reynolds WS, Patel R, Msezane L, et al. Current use of artificial urinary sphincters in the United States. J Urol. 2007;178:578–83.

39. Matsushita K, Chughtai BI, Maschino AC, et al. International variation in artificial urinary sphincter use. Urology. 2012;80:667–72.

40. Poon SA, Silberstein JL, Savage C, et al. Surgical practice patterns for male urinary incontinence: analysis of case logs from certifying American urologists. J Urol. 2012;188:205–10.

41. Kim PH, Pinheiro LC, Atoria CL, et al. Trends in the use of incontinence procedures after radical prostatectomy: a population based analysis. J Urol. 2013;189:602–8.

42. Lai HH, Boone TB. The surgical learning curve of artificial urinary sphincter implantation: implications for prosthetic training and referral. J Urol. 2013;189:1437–43.

43. Sandhu JS, Maschino AC, Vickers AJ. The surgical learning curve for artificial urinary sphincter procedures compared to typical surgeon experience. Eur Urol. 2011;60:1285–90.

44. Lee R, Te AE, Kaplan SA, et al. Temporal trends in adoption of and indications for the artificial urinary sphincter. J Urol. 2009;181:2622–7.

45. Almallah YZ, Grimsley SJS. A report of a regional service for post-prostatectomy urinary incontinence: a model for best practice? Ther Adv Urol. 2015;7:69–75.

46. Magera JS, Inman BA, Elliott DS. Does preoperative topical antimicrobial scrub reduce positive surgical site culture rates in men undergoing artificial urinary sphincter placement? J Urol. 2007;178:1328–32. discussion 1332.

47. Tanner J, Norrie P and Melen K. Preoperative hair removal to reduce surgical site infection. Cochrane Database Syst Rev. 2011;(11):CD004122.

48. Wolf JS, Bennett CJ, Dmochowski RR, et al. Best practice policy statement on urologic surgery antimicrobial prophylaxis. J Urol. 2008;179:1379–90.

49. Darouiche RO, Wall MJ, Itani KMF, et al. Chlorhexidine-alcohol versus povidone-iodine for surgical-site antisepsis. N Engl J Med. 2010;362:18–26.

50. Yeung LL, Grewal S, Bullock A, et al. A comparison of chlorhexidine-alcohol versus povidone-iodine for eliminating skin flora before genitourinary prosthetic surgery: a randomized controlled trial. J Urol. 2013;189:136–40.

51. Wilson SK, Delk JR, Henry GD, et al. New surgical technique for sphincter urinary control system using upper transverse scrotal incision. J Urol. 2003;169:261–4.

52. Henry GD, Graham SM, Cleves MA, et al. Perineal approach for artificial urinary sphincter implantation appears to control male stress incontinence better than the transscrotal approach. J Urol. 2008;179:1475–9. discussion 1479.

53. Costa P, Mottet N, Rabut B, et al. The use of an artificial urinary sphincter in women with type III incontinence and a negative Marshall test. J Urol. 2001;165:1172–6.

54. Marqués Queimadelos A, Abascal García R, Muruamendiaraz Fernández V, et al. [Artificial sphincter implantation in women with urinary incontinence using a combined abdomino-vaginal approach]. Arch Esp Urol. 1999;52:877–80.

55. Rouprêt M, Misraï V, Vaessen C, et al. Laparoscopic approach for artificial urinary sphincter implantation in women with intrinsic sphincter deficiency incontinence: a single-centre preliminary experience. Eur Urol. 2010;57:499–504.

56. Yates DR, Phé V, Rouprêt M, et al. Robot-assisted laparoscopic artificial urinary sphincter insertion in men with neurogenic stress urinary incontinence. BJU Int. 2013;111:1175–9.

57. Fournier G, Callerot P, Thoulouzan M, et al. Robotic-assisted laparoscopic implantation of artificial urinary sphincter in women with intrinsic sphincter deficiency incontinence: initial results. Urology. 2014;84:1094–8.

58. Biardeau X, Rizk J, Marcelli F, et al. Robot-assisted laparoscopic approach for artificial urinary sphincter implantation in 11 women with urinary stress incontinence: surgical technique and initial experience. Eur Urol. 2015;67:937–42.

59. Rothschild J, Chang Kit L, Seltz L, et al. Difference between urethral circumference and artificial urinary sphincter cuff size, and its effect on postoperative incontinence. J Urol. 2014;191:138–42.

60. Margreiter M, Farr A, Sharma V, et al. Urethral buttressing in patients undergoing artificial urinary sphincter surgery. J Urol. 2013;189:1777–81.

61. Simhan J, Morey AF, Singla N, et al. 3.5 cm Artificial urinary sphincter cuff erosion occurs predominantly in irradiated patients. J Urol. 2015;193:593–7.

62. O'Connor RC, Lyon MB, Guralnick ML, et al. Long-term follow-up of single versus double cuff artificial urinary sphincter insertion for the treatment of severe postprostatectomy stress urinary incontinence. Urology. 2008;71:90–3.

63. Vayleux B, Rigaud J, Luyckx F, et al. Female urinary incontinence and artificial urinary sphincter: study of efficacy and risk factors for failure and complications. Eur Urol. 2011;59:1048–53.

64. Mandron E, Bryckaert P-E, Papatsoris AG. Laparoscopic artificial urinary sphincter implantation for female genuine stress urinary incontinence: technique and 4-year experience in 25 patients. BJU Int. 2010;106:1194–8. discussion 1198.

65. Köhler TS, Benson A, Ost L, et al. Intentionally retained pressure-regulating balloon in artificial urinary sphincter revision. J Sex Med. 2013;10:2566–70.

66. Cefalu CA, Deng X, Zhao LC, et al. Safety of the "drain and retain" option for defunctionalized urologic prosthetic balloons and reservoirs during artificial urinary sphincter and inflatable penile prosthesis revision surgery: 5-year experience. Urology. 2013;82:1436–9.

67. Ashley RA, Husmann DA. Artificial urinary sphincters placed after posterior urethral distraction injuries in children are at risk for erosion. J Urol. 2007;178:1813–5.

68. Smith PJ, Hudak SJ, Scott JF, et al. Transcorporal artificial urinary sphincter cuff placement is associated with a higher risk of postoperative urinary retention. Can J Urol. 2013;20:6773–7.

69. Seideman CA, Zhao LC, Hudak SJ, et al. Is prolonged catheterization a risk factor for artificial urinary sphincter cuff erosion? Urology. 2013;82:943–6.

70. Magera JS, Elliott DS. Artificial urinary sphincter infection: causative organisms in a contemporary series. J Urol. 2008;180:2475–8.

71. Hajivassiliou CA. A review of the complications and results of implantation of the AMS artificial urinary sphincter. Eur Urol. 1999;35:36–44.

72. Elliott DS, Barrett DM. Mayo Clinic long-term analysis of the functional durability of the AMS 800 artificial urinary sphincter: a review of 323 cases. J Urol. 1998;159:1206–8.

73. Lai HH, Hsu EI, Teh BS, et al. 13 years of experience with artificial urinary sphincter implantation at Baylor College of Medicine. J Urol. 2007;177:1021–5.

74. Rozanski AT, Tausch TJ, Ramirez D, et al. Immediate urethral repair during explantation prevents stricture formation after artificial urinary sphincter cuff erosion. J Urol. 2014;192:442–6.

75. Kim SP, Sarmast Z, Daignault S, et al. Long-term durability and functional outcomes among patients with artificial urinary sphincters: a 10-year retrospective review from the University of Michigan. J Urol. 2008;179:1912–6.

76. Gousse AE, Madjar S, Lambert MM, et al. Artificial urinary sphincter for post-radical prostatectomy urinary incontinence: long-term subjective results. J Urol. 2001;166:1755–8.

77. Venn SN, Greenwell TJ, Mundy AR. The long-term outcome of artificial urinary sphincters. J Urol. 2000;164:702–6. discussion 706–707.

78. Jain R, Mitchell S, Laze J, et al. The effect of surgical intervention for stress urinary incontinence (UI) on post-prostatectomy UI during sexual activity. BJU Int. 2012;109:1208–12.

79. Linder BJ, de Cogain M, Elliott DS. Long-term device outcomes of artificial urinary sphincter reimplantation following prior explantation for erosion or infection. J Urol. 2014;191:734–8.

80. Bates A, Martin R, Terry T. Complications following artificial urinary sphincter placement after radical prostatectomy and radiotherapy: a meta-analysis. BJU Int. 2015.

81. Girinsky T. Effects of ionizing radiation on the blood vessel wall. J Mal Vasc. 2000;25:321–4.

82. Martins FE, Boyd SD. Artificial urinary sphincter in patients following major pelvic surgery and/or radiotherapy: are they less favorable candidates? J Urol. 1995;153:1188–93.

83. McGeady JB, McAninch JW, Truesdale MD, et al. Artificial urinary sphincter placement in compromised urethras and survival: a comparison of virgin, radiated and reoperative cases. J Urol. 2014;192:1756–61.

84. Ngninkeu BN, van Heugen G, di Gregorio M, et al. Laparoscopic artificial urinary sphincter in women for type III incontinence: preliminary results. Eur Urol. 2005;47:793–7. discussion 797.

85. Chung E, Cartmill RA. 25-year experience in the outcome of artificial urinary sphincter in the treatment of female urinary incontinence. BJU Int. 2010;106:1664–7.

86. Costa P, Poinas G, Ben Naoum K, et al. Long-term results of artificial urinary sphincter for women with type III stress urinary incontinence. Eur Urol. 2013;63:753–8.

Troubleshooting and Optimizing Outcomes After Artificial Urinary Sphincter

6

Gillian Stearns and Jaspreet S. Sandhu

The gold standard for male stress urinary incontinence has long been the artificial urinary sphincter (AUS). Efficacy and satisfaction rates are high as long as the AUS is functional [1, 2]. Various complications have been reported, including infection, erosion, device malfunction, and residual or recurrent incontinence, but if these are approached in a systematic fashion, patient satisfaction may be restored.

Infection

Device infection is a relatively rare occurrence, normally occurring at a median of 3.7 months after implantation, stabilizing after 48 months [3]. Contemporary series report infection rates between 0.5 and 10.6 % [2, 4]. Gram positive cocci are the most commonly seen bacteria. Patients present with fever, erythema, persistent pain over the prosthesis, fixation of the pump to the scrotal wall, purulent drainage from the wound, or exposed prosthesis [5, 6].

Traditional management involves immediate removal of the device followed by delayed replacement

G. Stearns, M.D.
Department of Urology, University of Vermont, Burlington, VT, USA

J.S. Sandhu, M.D. (✉)
Department of Surgery, Urology Service, Memorial Sloan Kettering Cancer Center, New York, NY, USA
e-mail: sandhuj@mskcc.org

of the AUS, typically at 3–6 months after explant. There have been small case series involving immediate replacement of artificial urinary sphincter after ensuring no erosion [5], but this is not the standard of care due to the fact that there appears to be no worsening of outcomes with delayed implantation. Removal of the AUS and its components is satisfactory to resolve the infection and patient's symptoms. Meticulous surgical technique, appropriate use of perioperative antibiotics, and antibiotic coating of the sphincter components are all efforts used to decrease erosion rates. Current American Urologic Association Guidelines recommend preoperative antibiotics to be given in all patients consisting of an aminoglycoside and a first/second generation cephalosporin or Vancomycin [7].

Erosion

Urethral cuff erosion typically presents with difficulty voiding, dysuria, and hematuria. Unless there has been a surgical technical error resulting in an unrecognized intraoperative cuff erosion, this is normally not seen in the immediate postoperative period, and usually occurs between 15 and 18 months [8, 9]. Diagnosis is made with cystoscopy, results of which reveal at least a part of the urethral cuff within the urethral lumen (see Fig. 6.1). Management consists of removal of the AUS and urethral catheter for 3 weeks. If the erosion is severe enough, urethroplasty at the time of explantation may be warranted [10].

© Springer International Publishing Switzerland 2016
J.S. Sandhu (ed.), *Urinary Dysfunction in Prostate Cancer*, DOI 10.1007/978-3-319-23817-3_6

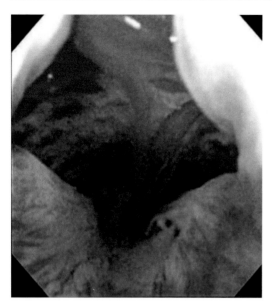

Fig. 6.1 Urethral cuff erosion seen for cystoscopy

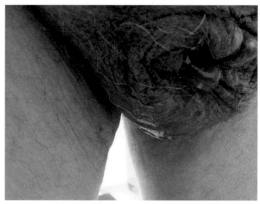

Fig. 6.2 Control pump eroded through scrotum

Urethral cuff erosion rates are highly variable, between 2 and 12 % in some series and depend on multiple factors [9, 11]. Patients at higher risk for erosion include those patients who have undergone radiation therapy, prior urethroplasty, multiple treatments for bladder neck contracture, urethral stent placement, or prior history of erosion/infection with a previous AUS. Higher explantation rates have been seen in those patients with prior infection/erosion, prior urethral stent, and those who had a 3.5 cm cuff [8, 11]. Some surgeons suggest that the higher rate of erosion with use of the 3.5 cm cuff may be due to a prior history of radiation, with 21 % of a radiated cohort experiencing erosion versus 4 % in those not radiated [12]. Prolonged urethral catheterization following AUS placement, defined as greater than 48 h, has also been associated with increased erosion rates [9]. Systemic disease states such as hypertension and coronary artery disease have been implicated as well, as these disease states portend vascular insufficiency, which may lead to tissue breakdown and ultimate cuff erosion [11]. While rare, pelvic or scrotal surgery for other causes might result in delayed erosion of the control pump, tubing, or reservoir (see Fig. 6.2). This scenario is managed just like an infected

artificial sphincter by explanting the entire device and re-implanting it 3–6 months later.

Erosion may be prevented by minimizing prolonged catheterization and urethral instrumentation, meticulous surgical technique, and delayed activation [9, 11]. Patient education is also important in helping to limit urethral instrumentation and prolonged catheterization. Patient brochures, wallet cards, and necklaces or bracelets with medical information help to prevent inadvertent urethral catheter placement prior to deactivation of the urethral cuff. Deactivating the cuff at intervals, especially at night, may help decrease rates of urethral erosion, and may be helpful in the high-risk patient [11].

Reimplantation of the sphincter usually occurs between 3 and 6 months post procedure [11, 13]. Follow-up cystoscopy is recommended prior to AUS replacement [11]. Some surgeons advocate for immediate urethral repair at the time of explantation, as urethral stricture may result at the site of erosion. Rates of stricture formation were found to be 38 % after in situ urethroplasty, as compared to 85 % in those managed with Foley catheter alone [13]. Transcorporal placement of at the time of AUS replacement may help in those patients who have had prior erosion. This has been repeatedly shown to be safe in patients with severely compromised urethras, including those with prior urethral insults [8]. Functional outcomes have been excellent, with 84 % of patients reporting 0-1 pad per day use [14].

However, it is associated with higher rates of postoperative erectile dysfunction and postoperative urinary retention [15]. Other alternatives have included urethral wrapping with xenograft such as small intestinal submucosa [16]. Although the case series are small, good functional outcomes have been reported [8, 16].

The 3.5 cm urethral cuff is the smallest and newest available cuff for the artificial urinary sphincter. The initial series by Hudak et al. showed similar explantation rates for erosion and infection for patients undergoing the 3.5 cm cuff in 67 patients. Most of these patients had undergone prior urethral surgeries and radiation [17]. The 3.5 cm cuff has been associated with higher erosion rates as previously mentioned in a recent prospective trial on multivariate analysis [8]. Those patients undergoing reimplantation following urethral erosion tend to have good continence outcomes, with over half reporting 0-1 pads daily [11]. However, these patients do have a fourfold higher rate of future erosion so patients must be counseled to this effect [11, 18].

Persistent or Recurrent Incontinence

Persistent or recurrent incontinence is a common presentation post-AUS to the urologist with multiple etiologies. Efficient and appropriate evaluation of the patient and device will help determine the next most effective modality of treatment.

Persistent Incontinence

In those patients that report immediate leakage after activation of the AUS, typically at the same level to that experienced prior to implantation, device malfunction—although rare this early—should be ruled out. If patients have irritative symptoms, hematuria, or signs of infection, then erosion should he high on the differential diagnosis. Other potential causes may include: improper operation of the pump, urinary tract infection,

occlusion of the tubing, or improper cuff sizing [19]. Improper operation results from a failure to fully deflate the cuff which may result in overflow incontinence. The pump may also be inadvertently deactivated by the patient, leading to persistent incontinence. If the pump is not placed in the proper location in the scrotum, the pump may be accidentally compressed while sitting, leading to unintentional cuff deflation [20]. Patient education is essential at the time of activation to help prevent this from occurring.

Detrusor overactivity or underactivity may appear de novo following prostatectomy. It may be associated with a urinary tract infection, and therefore urinalysis and urine culture may be helpful to rule out this as a potential source. Leach et al. noted only 40 % of patients had pure stress incontinence as the etiology of their post-prostatectomy incontinence. The remaining 60 % had some aspect of bladder dysfunction, which was aided with urodynamics [21]. The exact mechanism of action behind new onset changes in detrusor function is unknown. Chung et al. evaluated the urodynamics of 264 patients with bladder dysfunction following radical prostatectomy and noted detrusor underactivity in 108 (45 %). Minimally invasive prostatectomy was the only factor predictive of detrusor underactivity on univariate analysis [22]. Possible etiologies include decentralization of the bladder caused by mobilization at the time of prostatectomy, infection, inflammation or wall remodeling from fashioning the bladder neck at the time of anastomosis [23]. This may be evaluated with urodynamics after infectious sources have been ruled out. Anticholinergics may help to alleviate these symptoms if related to detrusor overactivity.

Improper sizing of the cuff frequently leads to decreased but persistent incontinence. This sizing tends to be related to surgeon experience, with a decrease in reoperative rates seen with a rising number of AUS performed annually. A study by Sandhu showed the risk of reoperation to be 24 % in those patients with five prior cases, decreasing to 10.7 % with those surgeons having performed more than 200 implants [24]. The pressure regulating balloon may also need to be evaluated to ensure that there is an appropriate level of fluid in the reservoir. Multiple techniques, including downsizing of the cuff, placement of a tandem cuff, placement of a transcorporal cuff, or placement of a higher pressure pressure-regulating balloon are available to improve persistent urinary incontinence. The decision to change just a component (e.g., just changing the urethral cuff when downsizing) versus replacing the entire device is dependent on time from initial implantation. Most authorities will replace the entire device with appropriate component modification if the initial device was placed more than 2 years prior.

Device Malfunction

Device malfunction rates increase with the life of the AUS. Clemens et al. noted a 50 % freedom from reoperative rate at 5 years with a cuff reoperative rate of 60 % in the same time period [2]. Another study showed a device survival rate of 66 % at 10 years [25]. The incidence of mechanical dysfunction has decreased significantly since the introduction of the narrow-back cuff in 1987, decreasing the rates from 21 % to 7.6 % in a single center study of 323 patients [4].

Device failure typically presents with sudden onset of recurrent urinary incontinence [6, 10]. Management of device failure is dependent on the time since AUS implantation. For failures soon after placement, other pathologies, such as bladder neck contracture, erosion, or bladder pathology should be ruled out. This is best done with cystoscopy. Once those etiologies have been ruled out, the sphincter itself should be evaluated. Ensuring that there are appropriate levels of fluid has been included in algorithms for troubleshooting previously, but there has been debate how to appropriately evaluate this [10]. Physical exam may reveal a pump that feels empty or cycles quickly; however, this has been shown to not be as sensitive as imaging [26]. Initially all AUS reservoirs were filled with dilute contrast and a plain-film abdominal X-ray was sufficient to evaluate the volume of the reservoir balloon. This remains an option according to the most recent AMS Operating Room Manual [26]. Injectable saline is now the preferred option for the filling of the AMS800 and renders plain-film X-ray ineffective for reservoir evaluation. Cross-sectional imaging is the current mainstay in noting the volume of fluid in the pressure regulating balloon. In particular, ultrasound has been reported to be useful and spares the patient radiation exposure that may be experienced with CT scan. Brucker et al. reported 100 % sensitivity when using office-based ultrasound to evaluate fluid volume [26]. If this is performed outside of the office setting, discussion with the radiologist is essential to ensure appropriate visualization and measurement of the reservoir. Figure 6.3 shows examples of formal limited pelvic ultrasounds performed to

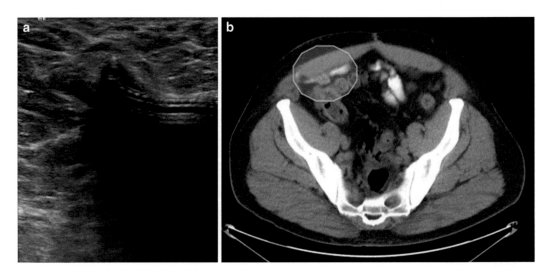

Fig. 6.3 (**a**) Limited pelvic ultrasound with deflated cuff; (**b**) CT scan showing deflated cuff (within *shaded oval*)

evaluate volume of the pressure-regulating balloon (Fig. 6.3 is an example of sonogram and CT scan with unfilled PRBs). A rough rule of thumb is that the diameter of the balloon should not be less than 3.8 cm, which corresponds roughly to 24 mL of fluid. Some practitioners advocate for use of electrical conductance testing to identify the faulty component and site of the leak at the time of operative revision [10, 20, 26].

In cases of device failure, the most common site of failure, defines as leak of urine on filling the component, is usually the urethral cuff. Some authorities will only replace the entire AUS device if the original was placed more than 3 years prior. Some practitioners will keep the pressure regulating balloon in place at the time of revision, placing a second reservoir on the contralateral side [27, 28]. They report a rate of infection similar to those with all components removed, 1.8 versus 1.5 %, respectively [27]. An ohmmeter has also been used to only revise the components with the leak [20]. However, if the leak is small, there may be false negative testing, resulting in the need for further revision. We advocate removing and replacing the entire device, regardless of when the initial device was placed, if there is a fluid leak in the system, diagnosed by imaging that demonstrates decreased amount of fluid in the pressure-regulating balloon. This is because of the fact that there has been, by definition, communication between the fluid within the hydraulic system of the artificial urinary sphincter and body fluids.

Idiopathic Leakage

Frequently patients will present to their urologist complaining of leakage after sitting on a hard stool for an extended period of time, resulting in embarrassing social incontinence, even in men who are otherwise dry. In an ex vivo study, extrinsic cuff compression resulted in reflux of dye back towards the pressure regulating balloon. After compression for 20 s, the pressure in the cuff decreased and urine was able to leak out [29]. The patient should be reassured that this is a normal occurrence and may find improved continence with the use of cushions and padded seats.

Urethral Strictures/Bladder Neck Contractures

The rate of anastomotic stricture after radical prostatectomy has been reported to be between 2.7–25.7 %, up to 62 % in those patients who undergo radiotherapy [30, 31]. In a study by Sandhu et al., anastomotic strictures were found to be associated with obesity, age, open surgical approach, renal insufficiency, and presence of a perioperative hematoma or urine leak [32]. In patients with a stricture following AUS placement, management can be difficult as instrumentation leads to an increased urethral erosion risk and the stricture causes bothersome symptoms and possible return of incontinence. Weissbart et al. reported a series of patients managed with Holmium YAG laser using a rigid ureteroscope. All patients had an anastomotic stricture prior to AUS that had been aggressively resected. Prior to AUS placement, cystoscopy was performed to ensure no recurrence. Mean time to repeat anastomotic stricture at 57 weeks and confirmed by office cystoscopy. Incisions were made at 3 and 9 o'clock with a 365 nm laser fiber [33]. Mark et al. recommended synchronous endoscopic treatment and out of 26 patients, only one recurred. His recurrent stricture was managed at the time of sphincter revision [34].

Success Rate of Revision Surgery

Secondary reimplantation has outcomes similar to those of virgin AUS placement. Reoperation rates were 17.5 in primary AUS cases versus 25 % in salvage AUS cases in a study by Linder et al. Salvage cases were performed for erosion, infection, or urethral atrophy. No difference was seen in 5-year survival rates (66 vs. 71 %, respectively). Median time to repeat explantation was 6 months [35]. Another group found that time to revision occurred at a median of 20.1 months. Of those patients undergoing revision, 44.7 % of patients did not require any further procedures. The most common indication for revision was recurrent incontinence. If the patient underwent explantation for erosion, 76.3 % of patients did not require a further procedure after reimplantation [36]. These patients post erosion do have a higher risk of erosion [11] and should be counseled for this at the time of reimplantation. Overall device outcomes (infection, atrophy, leaks, mechanical failure) were found to be no different from virgin cases [18].

Conclusions

The artificial urinary sphincter is a durable solution for treatment of stress urinary incontinence in the male resulting in high patient satisfaction. The management of AUS complications is reasonably straightforward and should be approached in a systematic fashion, resulting in improved efficiency in resolution of patient symptoms. Prevention of adverse outcomes is an area for future study.

References

1. Gousse AE, Madjar S, Lambert MM, Fishman IJ. Artificial urinary sphincter for post-prostatectomy incontinence: long-term subjective results. J Urol. 2001;166(5):1755–8.
2. Clemens JQ, Schuster TG, Konnak JW, McGuire EJ, Faerber GJ. Revision rate after artificial urinary sphincter implantation for incontinence after radical prostatectomy: actuarial analysis. J Urol. 2001; 166(4):1372–5.
3. Lai HH, Hsu EI, Teh BS, Butler EB, Boone TB. 13 years of experience with artificial urinary sphincter implantation at Baylor College of Medicine. J Urol. 2007;177(3):1021–5.
4. Elliott DS, Barrett DM. Mayo Clinic long-term analysis of the functional durability of the AMS 800 artificial urinary sphincter: a review of 323 cases. J Urol. 1998;159(4):1206–8.
5. Bryan DE, Mulcahy JJ, Simmons GR. Salvage procedure for infected noneroded artificial urinary sphincters. J Urol. 2002;168(6):2464–6.
6. Sandhu JS. Management of complications and residual symptoms in men with an artificial urinary sphincter. J Urol. 2014;192(2):303–4.
7. Wolf Jr JS, Bennett CJ, Dmochowski RR, Hollenbeck BK, Pearle MS, Schaeffer AJ, Urologic Surgery Antimicrobial Prophylaxis Best Practice Policy Panel. Best practice policy statement on urologic surgery antimicrobial prophylaxis. J Urol. 2008;179(4):1379–90.
8. Brant WO, Erickson BA, Elliott SP, Powell C, Alsikafi N, McClung C, Myers JB, Voelzke BB, Smith 3rd TG,

Broghammer JA. Risk factors for erosion of artificial urinary sphincters: a multicenter prospective study. Urology. 2014;84(4):934–8.
9. Seideman CA, Zhao LC, Hudak SJ, Mierzwiak J, Adibi M, Morey AF. Is prolonged catheterization a risk factor for artificial urinary sphincter cuff erosion? Urology. 2013;82(4):943–6.
10. Webster GD, Sherman ND. Management of male incontinence following artificial urinary sphincter failure. Curr Opin Urol. 2005;15(6):386–90.
11. Raj GV, Peterson AC, Toh KL, Webster GD. Outcomes following erosions of the artificial urinary sphincter. J Urol. 2006;175(6):2186–90.
12. Simhan J, Morey AF, Singla N, Tausch TJ, Scott JF, Lemack GE, Roehrborn CG. 3.5 cm Artificial urinary sphincter cuff erosion occurs predominantly in irradiated patients. J Urol. 2015;193(2):593–7.
13. Rozanski AT, Tausch TJ, Ramirez D, Simhan J, Scott JF, Morey AF. Immediate urethral repair during explantation prevents stricture formation after artificial urinary sphincter cuff erosion. J Urol. 2014; 192(2):442–6.
14. Guralnick ML, Miller E, Toh KL, Webster GD. Transcorporal artificial urinary sphincter cuff placement in cases requiring revision for erosion and urethral atrophy. J Urol. 2002;167(5):2075–8.
15. Smith PJ, Hudak SJ, Scott JF, Zhao LC, Morey AF. Transcorporal artificial urinary sphincter cuff placement is associated with a higher risk of postoperative urinary retention. Can J Urol. 2013;20(3):6773–7.
16. Rahman NU, Minor TX, Deng D, Lue TF. Combined external urethral bulking and artificial urinary sphincter for urethral atrophy and stress urinary incontinence. BJU Int. 2005;95(6):824–6.
17. Hudak SJ, Morey AF. Impact of 3.5 cm artificial urinary sphincter cuff on primary and revision surgery for male stress urinary incontinence. J Urol. 2011;186(5):1962–6.
18. Lai HH, Boone TB. Complex artificial urinary sphincter revision and reimplantation cases--how do they fare compared to virgin cases? J Urol. 2012; 187(3):951–5.
19. Furlow WL, Barrett DM. Recurrent or persistent urinary incontinence in patients with the artificial urinary sphincter: diagnostic considerations and management. J Urol. 1985;133(5):792–5.
20. Chung E, Cartmill R. Diagnostic challenges in the evaluation of persistent or recurrent urinary incontinence after artificial urinary sphincter (AUS) implantation in patients after prostatectomy. BJU Int. 2013;112 Suppl 2:32–5.
21. Leach GE, Trockman B, Wong A, Hamilton J, Haab F, Zimmern PE. Post-prostatectomy incontinence: urodynamic findings and treatment outcomes. J Urol. 1996;155(4):1256–9.
22. Chung DE, Dillon B, Kurta J, Maschino A, Cronin A, Sandhu JS. Detrusor underactivity is prevalent after radical prostatectomy: a urodynamic study including risk factors. Can Urol Assoc J. 2013;7(1-2):E33–7

23. Thiruchelvam N, Cruz F, Kirby M, Tubaro A, Chapple C, Sievert KD. A review of detrusor overactivity and the overactive bladder after radical prostate cancer treatment. BJU Int Forthcoming 2015

24. Sandhu JS, Maschino AC, Vickers AJ. The surgical learning curve for artificial urinary sphincter procedures compared to typical surgeon experience. Eur Urol. 2011;60(6):1285–90.

25. Venn SN, Greenwell TJ, Mundy AR. The long-term outcome of artificial urinary sphincters. J Urol. 2000;164:702–6.

26. AMS800 UrinaryControl Systemfor Male, Female and Pediatric Patients: Operating Room Manual. American Medical Systems, Inc; 2014

27. Brucker BM, Demirtas A, Fong E, Kelly C, Nitti VW. Artificial urinary sphincter revision: the role of ultrasound. Urology. 2013;82(6):1424–8.

28. Cefalu CA, Deng X, Zhao LC, Scott JF, Mehta S, Morey AF. Safety of the "drain and retain" option for defunctionalized urologic prosthetic balloons and reservoirs during artificial urinary sphincter and inflatable penile prosthesis revision surgery: 5-year experience. Urology. 2013;82(6):1436–9.

29. Köhler TS, Benson A, Ost L, Wilson SK, Brant WO. Intentionally retained pressure-regulating balloon in artificial urinary sphincter revision. J Sex Med. 2013;10(10):2566–70.

30. Beaugerie A, Phé V, Munbauhal G, Chartier-Kastler E, Mozer P. Artificial urinary sphincter AMS 800™ in males--can we explain residual leaks when sitting? J Urol. 2014;192(2):483–7.

31. Elliott SP, Meng MV, Elkin EP, McAninch JW, Duchane J, Carroll PR, CaPSURE Investigators. Incidence of urethral stricture after primary treatment for prostate cancer: data From CaPSURE. J Urol. 2007;178(2):529–34.

32. Sandhu JS, Gotto GT, Herran LA, Scardino PT, Eastham JA, Rabbani F. Age, obesity, medical comorbidities and surgical technique are predictive of symptomatic anastomotic strictures after contemporary radical prostatectomy. J Urol. 2011;185(6):2148–52.

33. Weissbart SJ, Chughtai B, Elterman D, Sandhu JS. Management of anastomotic stricture after artificial urinary sphincter placement in patients who underwent salvage prostatectomy. Urology. 2013; 82(2):476–9.

34. Mark S, Pérez LM, Webster GD. Synchronous management of anastomotic contracture and stress urinary incontinence following radical prostatectomy. J Urol. 1994;151(5):1202–4.

35. Linder BJ, de Cogain M, Elliott DS. Long-term device outcomes of artificial urinary sphincter reimplantation following prior explantation for erosion or infection. J Urol. 2014;191(3):734–8.

36. Wang R, McGuire EJ, He C, Faerber GJ, Latini JM. Long-term outcomes after primary failures of artificial urinary sphincter implantation. Urology. 2012;79(4):922–8.

Management of Vesicourethral Anastomotic Stricture

Yuka Yamaguchi, Lee C. Zhao, and Allen T. Morey

Introduction

Due to the widespread use of PSA as a marker for prostate cancer, and radical prostatectomy as a common treatment modality for prostate cancer, bladder neck contracture (BNC), also referred to as anastomotic stricture [1], has become a not infrequent cause of voiding dysfunction. The reported incidence of bladder neck contracture ranges widely from 0.4 to 32 % of patients [3, 2, 4]. Higher rates of 20–30 % tend to be reported in earlier reports (prior to the era of robotic assisted laparoscopic prostatectomy) [5–7, 10, 11]. Reports from the past decade indicate the rate of BNC after laparoscopic or robotic prostatectomy to be 4–6 % [9, 14]. The true incidence of bladder neck contracture, however, is unknown, as routine endoscopic evaluation is not performed in the majority of cases and diagnosis of BNC is largely dependent on presentation and evaluation of urinary symptoms [12]. Clearly, the presence of bladder neck contracture is a factor in patient satisfaction, as presence of BNC or urethral stricture was found on patient questionnaires to negatively affect a patient's willingness to undergo treatment again [6].

Risk Factors

Various factors have been associated with the formation of BNC, including surgeon specific, intraoperative, as well as patient specific factors [15, 16].

Surgeon volume has been demonstrated to affect rates of complications such as BNC after radical prostatectomy. Begg et al. evaluated data from the SEER-Medicare database and determined that higher volume surgeons were associated with a lower rate of post-prostatectomy urinary complications including anastomotic strictures [13]. In 2011, Sandhu et al. reported a single institution study in which the individual surgeon was a predictive factor in the occurrence of BNC [14]. They suggested that this reflected varying surgeon experience and skill as well as the varying technical approaches taken by the individual surgeons. Further, they demonstrated that surgical approach, laparoscopic versus open technique, was the strongest predictor of a symptomatic BNC with a hazard ratio of 0.11, $p < 0.0001$. Improved visualization with magnification during the construction of the anastomosis,

Y. Yamaguchi, M.D.
Department of Urology, NYU Langone Medical Center, New York, NY, USA

L.C. Zhao, M.D., M.S. (✉)
Department of Urology, New York University Langone Medical Center, 150 E 32nd St, 2nd Floor, New York, NY 10016, USA
e-mail: lee.zhao@nyumc.org

A.T. Morey, M.D.
Department of Urology, UT Southwestern Medical Center, Dallas, TX, USA

© Springer International Publishing Switzerland 2016
J.S. Sandhu (ed.), *Urinary Dysfunction in Prostate Cancer*, DOI 10.1007/978-3-319-23817-3_7

continuous suture technique, and overall decreased blood loss are all factors which have been suggested as reasons for decreased incidence of BNC with the minimally invasive technique. This echoed a previous report by Hu et al. that the minimally invasive approach had lower rates of anastomotic strictures than the open technique [9].

Intraoperative factors such as increased operative time and increased estimated blood loss have been associated with a higher risk of BNC [15]. A retrospective studies by Surya et al. identified urine leak and excessive blood loss as risk factors—complications which predispose to anastomotic leak and/or disruption. Sandhu et al. in a larger retrospective study demonstrated that urine leak and pelvic hematoma were independently associated with the symptomatic BNCs. However, Levy et al. reported that contrast extravasation on voiding cystourethrogram at 3 weeks did not increase risk of BNC [16].

Patient characteristics contributing to BNC include cigarette smoking, diabetes, CAD, HTN, obesity, and age. Analysis of data from the Cancer of the Prostate Strategic Urologic Research Endeavor (CapSURE) database demonstrated that age older than 70 years and obesity were strong predictors of the need for stricture related treatment after prostate cancer therapy [8]. This study in particular did not differentiate between urethral strictures and bladder neck contractures. However, a study from Memorial Sloan Kettering Cancer Center also demonstrated age and BMI are independent factors associated with symptomatic bladder neck contractures, specifically [14]. Obesity was previously associated with higher pathological Gleason grade, higher positive surgical margin rates, higher risk of tumor recurrence [8]. It is hypothesized that obesity may cause technical difficulties in performing a good anastomosis with mucosa to mucosa apposition and may poorly influence healing [8].

Further, Sandhu et al. found that Charlson comorbidity index was associated with development of symptomatic vesicourethral anastomotic stricture [14]. Specific comorbid factors that have been reported to be associated with a higher incidence of BNC include coronary artery disease (CAD), hypertension (HTN), and diabetes (DM), renal disease, and history of cigarette smoking [14, 15]. All these risk factors suggest the effect of microvascular disease on wound healing

Park et al. reported that bladder neck contracture was associated with increased post-prostatectomy scar width greater than 10 mm and hypothesized that BNC may be related to a hypertrophic scarring mechanism [17]. Prior TURP has been also identified as a risk factor [18]. Radiation status is also a significant risk factor, both in the primary and adjuvant setting. The use of external beam radiation after radical prostatectomy has been shown to increase the risk of BNC [8]. Patients undergoing salvage prostatectomy after radiation also have an eight-fold increased probability (47.0 vs. 5.8) of BNC than those undergoing standard radical prostatectomy [19]. Radiation not only increases the probability of BNC but also tends to make them more difficult to treat. A greater average number of procedures were needed to stabilize BNC in the salvage prostatectomy than in the standard radical prostatectomy group, including 1.24 vs. 1.15 dilatations, 0.88 vs. 0.58 incisions and 0.71 vs. 0.08 resections [19].

Presentation

Evaluation of the CapSURE database has demonstrated that most post-prostatectomy strictures present within the first 6 months after radical prostatectomy with a decreasing incidence through the subsequent 2 years, while radiation strictures occur with increasing frequency through the first 4 years of follow-up [8].

Patients present with obstructive urinary symptoms including decreased urinary stream, dribbling, nocturia, incomplete voiding, or even complete retention [20]. Many also have incontinence. Multivariate analysis has demonstrated that BNC is an independent risk factor for urinary incontinence after radical prostatectomy [21]. BNC may have several effects on continence. Outlet obstruction may worsen any component of bladder overactivity, increasing urge incontinence. BNC may also mask underlying sphincteric deficiency and thus treatment of the contracture may worsen continence [1]. On the other hand according to some authors, scarring of the outlet may prevent adequate coaptation of preserved external sphincters and thus treatment of the bladder neck contracture may improve continence [22].

Clearly a certain unknown percentage of patients remain asymptomatic and undiagnosed or are only diagnosed incidentally, for instance, upon inability to catheterize for an unrelated surgical procedure [12].

Evaluation

Evaluation may include midstream urinalysis and urine culture to ensure the absence of infection. Uroflowmetry may reveal a decreased Qmax with an obstructive pattern. There may be incomplete emptying of the bladder with elevated post void residual. Cystoscopic evaluation demonstrates well defined annular scar at the level of the urethrovesical anastomosis (Fig. 7.1), below the bladder neck and proximal to the membranous urethra and the sphincter complex [23]. The severity of BNC may range from a slight narrowing of the lumen preventing passage of the cysto-

scope (Fig. 7.1) to complete obliteration (Fig. 7.2). However if the scar is not yet mature, as may occur in patients who are less than 8 weeks after prostatectomy, the area of scar may be poorly defined [20]. Retrograde urethrogram and voiding cystourethrogram may be used to delineate stricture anatomy. In cases of obliterative contractures, the patient will need a suprapubic catheter for urinary drainage. Subsequently, antegrade cystoscopy through the suprapubic tract can be performed to accurately identify the proximal extent of the obliterated segment, while retrograde urethroscopy can delineate the distal extent of the stricture.

This evaluation is generally sufficient for a clear-cut case of obstructive urinary symptoms and a cystoscopic evidence of anastomotic contracture. However, if there is concomitant stress or urge urinary incontinence urodynamic testing allows assessment of bladder overactivity and recruitment of abdominal musculature for voiding [24].

Management

Several authors have described algorithms for treatment of BNCs which generally progress from less invasive endoscopic management to

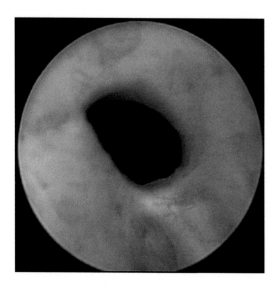

Fig. 7.1 Typical appearance of a bladder neck contracture on cystoscopic evaluation. There is a well defined annular scar at the level of the urethrovesical anastomosis

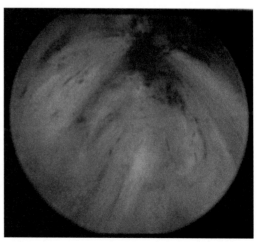

Fig. 7.2 Bladder neck contractures may also be obliterative. There is no visible lumen on cystoscopic evaluation of this bladder neck

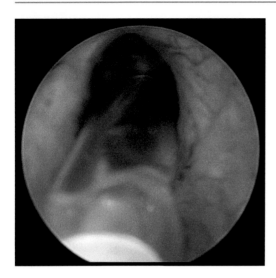

Fig. 7.3 This is the cystoscopic appearance of a balloon dilator passing through a bladder neck contracture

open reconstruction [25, 26]. Management may include simple dilation, optical internal bladder neck incision, transurethral resection of the stricture and finally open surgical reconstruction of the bladder neck.

Initial management of BNC is generallyure-thral dilation. A single dilation or urethrotomy successfully manages BNC in 24–73 % of patients [15]. This may be performed by filiform and followers, Van Buren sounds, or balloon dilation in the office (Fig. 7.3) [20, 27]. Some authors have favored balloon dilation for initial treatment of BNC [28, 29]. Ramchandani et al. reported a 59 % success rate with initial balloon dilation with no subsequent urinary incontinence. Serial dilation may be combined with a schedule of self-catheterization to maintain bladder outlet patency [17, 25]. Park et al. reported a regimen using dilation with Nottingham dilators to 18 French followed by a 3 month self-dilation regimen [17]. 73.1 % of the patients were success-fully managed with this regimen with one or two dilations followed by self-catheterization. However, dilations are uncomfortable for patients, may cause trauma to the bladder neck, and may be a source of infections. Furthermore, patients with urethral strictures performing self-catheterization have been reported to have a sig-nificant decrease in quality of life [30]. Moreover

in patients with concomitant incontinence who may need AUS placement, intermittent catheter-ization should be avoided due to concern for ero-sion. Thus, other options for management of refractory BNC are desired.

More aggressive intervention with bladder neck incision or bladder neck resection has been suggested for refractory BNC [18, 20, 27]. Generally, bladder neck incision involves inci-sion of the scar at 3, 9, and in some instances, the 6 o'clock position. There is some variation based on surgeon preference. However, the optimal modality for transurethral incision of bladder neck is unknown.

Cold knife urethrotomy has success rates as high as 25–87 % for uncomplicated cases [27]. Dalkin et al. advocated for urethrotomy using the cold knife urethrotome at the 4 o'clock and 8 o'clock positions at the level of the scar down to bleeding tissue [20, 24]. Foley catheter was left for 72 h after the urethrotomy. If the scar appeared immature at initial presentation, they recom-mended initial dilation with filiform and followers followed by urethrotomy once the scar was mature. The same group later reported their long term fol-low-up: at a mean follow-up of 30 months, repeat urethrotomies were required in 17 % of patients [24]. Using a continence questionnaire they estab-lished that continence rates between the urethrot-omy patients and control patients were also not statistically different. Cold knife urethrotomy may be used as a primary treatment or secondary treat-ment when dilation fails.

Electrocautery or "hot" knife incision has also been used for bladder neck incisions generally have been used for denser strictures refractory to prior endoscopic management. Ramirez et al. reported a technique in which intraoperative bal-loon dilation of the BNC is followed by deep lat-eral incisions with Collings knife at 3 and 9 o'clock (Figs. 7.4 and 7.5) [26]. This allows pas-sage of the resectoscope proximal to the bladder neck prior to performing bladder neck incisions, which allows incisions to be directly visualized and incised deeply. Most of their patients (78 %) were refractory to prior endoscopic management. The authors reported a 72 % success rate on ini-tial TUIBNC at a mean follow-up of 12.9 months.

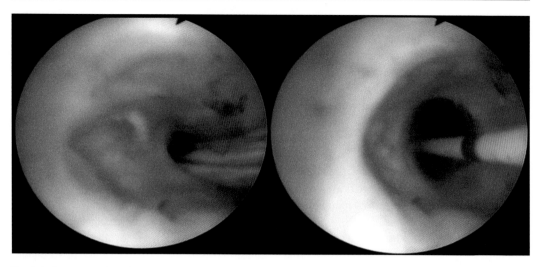

Fig. 7.4 Demonstration of intraoperative balloon dilation of the bladder neck contracture. The balloon dilator is passed over a wire through the bladder neck contracture and then is inflated

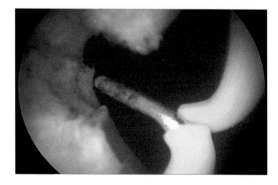

Fig. 7.5 Balloon dilation of the bladder neck contracture allows passage of the resectoscope into the bladder. The bladder neck contracture is further opened using deep lateral incisions with Collings knife at 3 and 9 o'clock

Laser urethrotomy has been advocated due to ability to achieve precise incisions and achieve hemostasis [31, 32]. In particular, the Ho:YAG laser is thought to be advantageous for urethrotomy due to its shallow tissue absorption of less than 0.5 mm [25]. This minimizes the effect of the laser on surrounding tissue thus decreasing the risk of scar formation. Lagerveld et al. used Ho:YAG laser to make a deep incision at the bladder neck at 6 o'clock followed by vaporization of scar tissue from the 3 to 9 o'clock positions in 10 patients. At a mean follow-up of 18 months (range 3–29 months) no patients needed treatment for restenosis. Other authors reported the use of the Ho:YAG laser for BNC refractory to multiple prior endoscopic interventions [32]. While the number of patients in this case series was small (three), they reported successful treatment at a follow-up of 11–37 months.

Transurethral resection of bladder neck has been suggested for longer strictures resistant to other endoscopic intervention [33]. However, the risk of incontinence is may be high [18]. Surya et al. found that three of four patients undergoing bladder neck resection had subsequent incontinence. Popken et al. conversely reported successful resection of scar without incurring increased risk of incontinence [23].

Several different techniques have been suggested when the vesicourethral junction is obliterated. Combined antegrade and retrograde recanalization with a stiff guide wire has been used with various modalities including cold knife, electrocautery and laser used to core out the lumen [34, 35]. Carr and Webster described a technique in which a sternal wire was guided from the urethra into the area of the bladder neck under vision via antegrade cystoscopy. Once the wire was in the correct location, cold knife incisions were used to regain urethrovesical continuity. While all four patients were able to regain urethrovesical continuity, three of the four patients required self catheterizations to maintain patency for the long term.

Roughly one-third of BNCs may be refractory to three or more attempts at endoscopic treatment [15]. Given the difficulty in managing refractory BNCs, some have advocated combining bladder neck incision with injection therapy with antiproliferative agents such as triamcinolone or mitomycin [36, 37]. Eltahawy et al. reported a technique in which holmium laser was used to perform transurethral incision of the bladder neck with subsequent injection of triamcinolone at the incision sites. They reported a 83 % success rate at a mean follow-up of 24 months (range 6–72 months) [36].

Mitomycin C has also been used as an adjunct to internal urethrotomy for recalcitrant BNC [37]. The Lahey clinic reported a technique in which cold knife incisions of bladder neck were performed followed by injection of mitomycin C. At a median follow-up of 12 months, 72 % of the patients had a stable, open bladder neck after one procedure; 22 % of patients required repeat procedures to stabilize their bladder neck.

Some authors have advocated endoscopic management coupled with placement of permanent intraurethal stents (UroLume™) in BNCs resistant to endoscopic management only [7, 25]. The UroLume™ Wallstent was a stainless steam tubed mesh which allows for epithelial ingrowth, theoretically preventing migration, infection, and encrustation, which was initially reported on the use for urethral strictures by Milroy [38]. The placement of the UroLume stent interfered with sphincter function and thus jeopardized continence; therefore several authors advocated with UroLume™ placement at the bladder neck followed by artificial urinary sphincter placement. There are well known complications: stent migration, perineal pain, hematuria, stent encrustation, and growth of obstructive hyperplastic tissue [39, 40]. However, initial studies reported a high success rate with one study reporting a 89 % patient satisfaction rate at a mean follow-up of 17.5 months [40]. Anger et al. reported the UroLume as a reasonable option to offer patients with recurrent BNC to avoid chronic indwelling catheter or more invasive options such as urinary diversion or open reconstruction [25]. However, longer follow-up has revealed a high rate of com-

plications [41, 42] with Magera et al. reporting a much lower success rate of 52 % at initial stent insertion [43]. Erickson et al. reported a 53 % stent specific reoperation rate [42] and suggested that stents only be offered in patients who did not desire or were medically unfit for open reconstruction. The UroLume stent is no longer commercially available in the United States.

Open Repair

When above treatments fail, the patient should be considered for revision of the vesicourethral anastomosis if they are medically fit to endure surgery. Multiple attempts at endoscopic management may result in complex dense, long, or obliterative strictures. Existing reports of revisions of vesicourethral anastomosis are from high volume reconstruction centers and abdomino-perineal, transpubic, and transperineal approaches have been described [12, 29, 44]. Incontinence after anastomotic revision is the norm rather than the exception and a plan for management of incontinence, whether in synchronous or staged fashion, should be in place.

The transperineal approach start with a perineal incision for mobilization of the urethra up to the level of stricture where the urethra is transected and all scar tissue is excised until only healthy tissue remains. Maneuvers such as separation of the crura or inferior pubectomy may be performed to allow access to the bladder neck. Mundy and Andrich prefer a strictly transperineal approach and reported success in 88 % of the patients without a history of radiation [12]. The remaining patients underwent a second revision with good results. Of note, radiation decreased success rates substantially to 66 %. All reconstructed patients subsequently required AUS placement.

Simonato et al. described a "pull through" method using a combined perineal and suprapubic approach [45]. In this approach, after the urethra is mobilized perineally, the bladder is punctured suprapubically and the tract dilated to accommodate an Amplatz sheath. The suprapubic access is then used to insert a sound over a guidewire into the bladder neck which identifies the proximal extent of stricture. Once the strictured segment is excised and the urethra prepared, sutures placed on the proximal stump of the urethra are pulled into the bladder neck via the suprapubic access. A catheter is placed and sutures are placed in the paraurethral fascia and vesicourethral anastomosis to create a watertight anastomosis. Ten out of 11 patients required AUS placement 6 month after their bladder neck reconstruction for complete incontinence.

Theodorou et al. described their abdomino-perineal approach in which an abdominal incision is made in addition to the perineal incision to assist with mobilization of the bladder and urethra from above [46]. Scar was excised from both perineal and abdominal approaches. The bladder was mobilized from the abdominal incision and advanced to meet the urethra, which was brought in from the perineal route. Concomitant ileocystoplasty was performed if required, for bladder overactivity resistant to medical treatment. All patients underwent simultaneous AUS placement. At mean follow-up of 24.42 months, five patients were able to void well without obstruction while one patient required clean intermittent catheterization to empty his augmented bladder.

Wessells et al. described the experience at the University of California, San Francisco (UCSF) and emphasized the need for an approach tailored to the anatomy of the individual patient [44]. They described varied approaches in four patients with BNC refractory to endoscopic management. One was an abdomino-perineal approach where the urethra was mobilized perineally but a cystotomy was necessary to appropriately visualize the anastomotic suture placement. While the perineal approach is similar to urethroplasty for posterior urethral disruption, prior prostatectomy causes fibrotic changes that make the bladder less mobile than in posterior urethral disruption, necessitating the additional abdominal approach for bladder mobilization in select cases [44]. Pubectomy was performed in two patients, one in whom a urethropubic sinus required excision and another in whom pubectomy facilitated exposure for the formation of a bladder tube to anastomose to the urethra. In an update of their experience,

they suggested that pubectomy was helpful in strictures longer than 2 cm [47]. One patient had a long stricture from radiation, salvage prostatectomy, and multiple endoscopic interventions. He underwent a reconstruction via a perineal approach with a penile fasciocutaneous flap ventral onlay. The varied approaches for each patient emphasize the need to tailor treatment to the individual.

In the majority of vesicourethral anastomosis revisions, incontinence is expected. However, there have been reports of BNC repairs with preservation of continence, albeit on a small number of patients. Schlossberg et al. reported reconstruction in two patients using a combined abdominal and perineal approach, partial pubectomy, and omental wrap around the new anastomosis [29]. Both patients were continent post operatively; the authors maintain that continent vesicourethral reconstruction is possible if the membranous urethra remains functionally intact. Chiou et al. reported a novel technique of endo-urethroplasty in which a meshed preputial skin graft is placed via a catheter [48]. Initially multiple bladder neck incisions are made with a urethrotome. A Foley catheter is placed for 3–5 days until the second stage in which a pediatric resectoscope is used to expose the granulation bed. A meshed preputial skin graft is placed around the Foley catheter and tacked into place via a suture passed through the urethra from the perineum. They have reported success on two patients while maintaining continence at 11 and 25-month follow-up.

Diversion

The last resort for treatment of recalcitrant bladder neck contracture, when outlet reconstruction fails, is urinary diversion. Chronic catheter drainage or suprapubic tube may be elected depending on patient preference and health status. However, if the bladder is of reasonable capacity, then a catheterizable limb may be created [33, 49]. In patients with prior radiation, evaluation with urodynamics is paramount to evaluate bladder capacity, compliance and overactivity to ensure simultaneous bladder augmentation is not required. Cystectomy with urinary diversion may also be appropriate if bladder function is poor.

Conclusion

BNC is an uncommon complication after radical prostatectomy that has been associated with a history of smoking and radiation therapy. While the majority of men with BNC can be managed with endoscopic treatment, recalcitrant bladder neck contractures present a complex problem requiring careful consideration of each patient's anatomy. Treatment of bladder neck contractures are often associated with incontinence which can be managed with an AUS after stabilization of the bladder outlet.

References

1. King T, Almallah YZ. Post-radical-prostatectomy urinary incontinence: the management of concomitant bladder neck contracture. Adv Urol. 2012;2012:295798.
2. Lange PH, Reddy PK. Technical nuances and surgical results of radical retropubic prostatectomy in 150 patients. J Urol. 1987;138(2):348–52.
3. Middleton AW. Pelvic lymphadenectomy with modified radical retropubic prostatectomy as a single operation: technique used and results in 50 consecutive cases. J Urol. 1981;125(3):353–6.
4. Davidson PJ, van den Ouden D, Schroeder FH. Radical prostatectomy: prospective assessment of mortality and morbidity. Eur Urol. 1996;29(2):168–73.
5. Fowler FJ, Barry MJ, Lu-Yao G, Roman A, Wasson J, Wennberg JE. Patient-reported complications and follow-up treatment after radical prostatectomy. The National Medicare Experience: 1988-1990 (updated June 1993). Urology. 1993;42(6):622–9.
6. Kao TC, Cruess DF, Garner D, Foley J, Seay T, Friedrichs P, et al. Multicenter patient self-reporting questionnaire on impotence, incontinence and stricture after radical prostatectomy. J Urol. 2000;163(3):858–64.
7. Erickson BA, Meeks JJ, Roehl KA, Gonzalez CM, Catalona WJ. Bladder neck contracture after retropubic radical prostatectomy: incidence and risk factors from a large single-surgeon experience. BJU Int. 2009;104(11):1615–9.
8. Elliott SP, Meng MV, Elkin EP, McAninch JW, Duchane J, Carroll PR, et al. Incidence of urethral stricture after primary treatment for prostate cancer: data From CaPSURE. J Urol. 2007;178(2):529–34. discussion 534.
9. Hu JC, Gu X, Lipsitz SR, Barry MJ, D'Amico AV, Weinberg AC, et al. Comparative effectiveness of minimally invasive vs open radical prostatectomy. JAMA. 2009;302(14):1557–64.
10. Breyer BN, Davis CB, Cowan JE, Kane CJ, Carroll PR. Incidence of bladder neck contracture after robot-assisted laparoscopic and open radical prostatectomy. BJU Int. 2010;106(11):1734–8.
11. Williams SB, Prasad SM, Weinberg AC, Shelton JB, Hevelone ND, Lipsitz SR, et al. Trends in the care of radical prostatectomy in the United States from 2003 to 2006. BJU Int. 2011;108(1):49–55.
12. Mundy AR, Andrich DE. Posterior urethral complications of the treatment of prostate cancer. BJU Int. 2012;110(3):304–25.
13. Begg CB, Riedel ER, Bach PB, Kattan MW, Schrag D, Warren JL, et al. Variations in morbidity after radical prostatectomy. N Engl J Med. 2002;346(15):1138–44.
14. Sandhu JS, Gotto GT, Herran LA, Scardino PT, Eastham JA, Rabbani F. Age, obesity, medical comorbidities and surgical technique are predictive of symptomatic anastomotic strictures after contemporary radical prostatectomy. J Urol. 2011;185(6):2148–52.
15. Borboroglu PG, Sands JP, Roberts JL, Amling CL. Risk factors for vesicourethral anastomotic stricture after radical prostatectomy. Urology. 2000;56(1):96–100.
16. Levy JB, Ramchandani P, Berlin JW, Broderick GA, Wein AJ. Vesicourethral healing following radical prostatectomy: is it related to surgical approach? Urology. 1994;44(6):888–92.
17. Park R, Martin S, Goldberg JD, Lepor H. Anastomotic strictures following radical prostatectomy: insights into incidence, effectiveness of intervention, effect on continence, and factors predisposing to occurrence. Urology. 2001;57(4):742–6.
18. Surya BV, Provet J, Johanson KE, Brown J. Anastomotic strictures following radical prostatectomy: risk factors and management. J Urol. 1990;143(4):755–8.
19. Gotto GT, Yunis LH, Vora K, Eastham JA, Scardino PT, Rabbani F. Impact of prior prostate radiation on complications after radical prostatectomy. J Urol. 2010;184(1):136–42.
20. Dalkin BL. Endoscopic evaluation and treatment of anastomotic strictures after radical retropubic prostatectomy. J Urol. 1996;155(1):206–8.
21. Eastham JA, Kattan MW, Rogers E, Goad JR, Ohori M, Boone TB, et al. Risk factors for urinary incontinence after radical prostatectomy. J Urol. 1996;156(5):1707–13.
22. Giannarini G, Manassero F, Mogorovich A, Valent F, De Maria M, Pistolesi D, et al. Cold-knife incision of anastomotic strictures after radical retropubic prostatectomy with bladder neck preservation: efficacy and impact on urinary continence status. Eur Urol. 2008;54(3):647–56.

23. Popken G, Sommerkamp H, Schultze-Seemann W, Wetterauer U, Katzenwadel A. Anastomotic stricture after radical prostatectomy. Incidence, findings and treatment. Eur Urol. 1998;33(4):382–6.
24. Yurkanin JP, Dalkin BL, Cui H. Evaluation of cold knife urethrotomy for the treatment of anastomotic stricture after radical retropubic prostatectomy. J Urol. 2001;165(5):1545–8.
25. Anger JT, Raj GV, Delvecchio FC, Webster GD. Anastomotic contracture and incontinence after radical prostatectomy: a graded approach to management. J Urol. 2005;173(4):1143–6.
26. Ramirez D, Zhao LC, Bagrodia A, Scott JF, Hudak SJ, Morey AF. Deep lateral transurethral incisions for recurrent bladder neck contracture: promising 5-year experience using a standardized approach. Urology. 2013;82(6):1430–5.
27. Breyer BN, McAninch JW. Management of recalcitrant bladder neck contracture after radical prostatectomy for prostate cancer. Endoscopic and open surgery. J Urol. 2011;185(2):390–1.
28. Ramchandani P, Banner MP, Berlin JW, Dannenbaum MS, Wein AJ. Vesicourethral anastomotic strictures after radical prostatectomy: efficacy of transurethral balloon dilation. Radiology. 1994;193(2):345–9.
29. Schlossberg S, Jordan G, Schellhammer P. Repair of obliterative vesicourethral stricture after radical prostatectomy: A technique for preservation of continence. Urology. 1995;45(3):510–3.
30. Lubahn JD, Zhao LC, Scott JF, Hudak SJ, Chee J, Terlecki R, et al. Poor quality of life in patients with urethral stricture treated with intermittent self-dilation. J Urol. 2014;191(1):143–7.
31. Lagerveld BW, Laguna MP, Debruyne FMJ, De La Rosette JJMCH. Holmium:YAG laser for treatment of strictures of vesicourethral anastomosis after radical prostatectomy. J Endourol. 2005;19(4):497–501.
32. Hayashi T, Yoshinaga A, Ohno R, Ishii N, Watanabe T, Yamada T, et al. Successful treatment of recurrent vesicourethral stricture after radical prostatectomy with holmium laser: report of three cases. Int J Urol. 2005;12(4):414–6.
33. Westney OL. Salvage surgery for bladder outlet obstruction after prostatectomy or cystectomy. Curr Opin Urol. 2008;18(6):570–4.
34. Carr LK, Webster GD. Endoscopic management of the obliterated anastomosis following radical prostatectomy. J Urol. 1996;156(1):70–2.
35. Dogra PN, Nabi G. Core-through urethrotomy using the neodymium: YAG laser for obliterative urethral strictures after traumatic urethral disruption and/or distraction defects: long-term outcome. J Urol. 2002;167(2 Pt 1):543–6.
36. Eltahawy E, Gur U, Virasoro R, Schlossberg SM, Jordan GH. Management of recurrent anastomotic stenosis following radical prostatectomy using hol-
mium laser and steroid injection. BJU Int. 2008;102(7):796–8.
37. Vanni AJ, Zinman LN, Buckley JC. Radial urethrotomy and intralesional mitomycin C for the management of recurrent bladder neck contractures. J Urol. 2011;186(1):156–60.
38. Milroy EJ, Chapple C, Eldin A, Wallsten H. A new treatment for urethral strictures: a permanently implanted urethral stent. J Urol. 1989;141(5):1120–2.
39. Corujo M, Badlani GH. Epithelialization of permanent stents. J Endourol Endourol Soc. 1997;11(6):477–80.
40. Elliott DS, Boone TB. Combined stent and artificial urinary sphincter for management of severe recurrent bladder neck contracture and stress incontinence after prostatectomy: a long-term evaluation. J Urol. 2001;165(2):413–5.
41. Anger J. Management of recalcitrant bladder neck contracture after radical prostatectomy for prostate cancer. UroLume stent. J Urol. 2011;185(2):391–2.
42. Erickson BA, McAninch JW, Eisenberg ML, Washington SI, Breyer BN. Management for prostate cancer treatment related posterior urethral and bladder neck stenosis with stents. J Urol. 2011;185(1):198–203.
43. Magera Jr JS, Inman BA, Elliott DS. Outcome analysis of urethral wall stent insertion with artificial urinary sphincter placement for severe recurrent bladder neck contracture following radical prostatectomy. J Urol. 2009;181(3):1236–41.
44. Wessells H, Morey AF, McAninch JW. Obliterative vesicourethral strictures following radical prostatectomy for prostate cancer: reconstructive armamentarium. J Urol. 1998;160(4):1373–5.
45. Simonato A, Gregori A, Lissiani A, Varca V, Carmignani G. Use of Solovov-Badenoch principle in treating severe and recurrent vesico-urethral anastomosis stricture after radical retropubic prostatectomy: technique and long-term results. BJU Int. 2012;110(11 Pt B):E456–60.
46. Theodoros C, Katsifotis C, Stournaras P, Moutzouris G, Katsoulis A, Floratos D. Abdomino-perineal repair of recurrent and complex bladder neck-prostatic urethra contractures. Eur Urol. 2000;38(6):734–40. discussion 740–1.
47. Elliott SP, McAninch JW, Chi T, Doyle SM, Master VA. Management of severe urethral complications of prostate cancer therapy. J Urol. 2006;176(6 Pt 1):2508–13.
48. Chiou RK, Howe S, Morton JJ, Grune MT, Taylor RJ. Treatment of recurrent vesicourethral anastomotic stricture after radical prostatectomy with endourethroplasty. Urology. 1996;47(3):422–5.
49. Castellan MA, Gosalbez R, Labbie A, Monti PR. Clinical applications of the Monti procedure as a continent catheterizable stoma. Urology. 1999;54(1):152–6.

Rectourethral Fistula

8

Jack M. Zuckerman and Kurt A. McCammon

Abbreviations

RUF	Rectourethral fistula
RP	Radical prostatectomy
EBRT	External beam radiation therapy
XRT	Radiation therapy
TURP	Transurethral resection of the prostate
HIFU	High-intensity focused ultrasound
CT	Computed tomography
MRI	Magnetic resonance imaging
RUG	Retrograde urethrogram
VCUG	Voiding cystourethrogram
BMG	Buccal mucosa graft
SPT	Suprapubic tube

Introduction

Rectourethral fistula (RUF) is a congenital or acquired abnormal communication between rectal and urethral epithelium. Congenital fistulas include those that occur in conjunction with anorectal malformations and are usually corrected at the time of pediatric anoplasty. Acquired fistulas may develop secondary to iatrogenic surgical

J.M. Zuckerman, M.D. • K.A. McCammon, M.D., F.A.C.S. (✉)
Department of Urology, Eastern Virginia Medical School, Norfolk, VA, USA
e-mail: MccammKA@EVMS.EDU

injury, trauma, infection/inflammation, malignancy, or tissue ablation [1]. Today, although rare, acquired fistulas most often result from complications of prostate cancer treatment. PSA testing has led to an increase in prostate cancer diagnosis and treatment over the last several decades. Multimodality therapy and tissue ablative techniques are also being performed with increasing frequency, leading to higher rates of RUF. While surgical fistulas are often small and uncomplicated, fistulas associated with radiation and/or tissue ablation are frequently larger with poorly vascularized tissues leading to more difficult repairs with poorer outcomes.

Etiology and Pathophysiology

The risk for rectal injury during radical prostatectomy (RP) is small and only a subset of these injuries will develop into an iatrogenic RUF. Thomas and colleagues published that the incidence RUF formation is 0.53 % (12/2447) following open radical prostatectomy [2]. The risk for fistula formation was higher in perineal (1.04 %) versus retropubic prostatectomy (0.34 %). Of these men, only 54 % of them were known to have an incidental rectal injury during prostatectomy, which was repaired at the time in two layers. Sixty-two percent of the men had extracapsular disease, suggesting either adherence to the rectal mucosa or surgeon attempts at wide local excision contributed to fistula formation. Robotic-assisted laparoscopic techniques appear to have even lower rates of rectal injury and fistula formation, though no direct comparisons can be made. Wedmid et al. published a series of 6650 robotic prostatectomies performed at six institutions [3]. They found only 11 rectal injuries (0.17 %), of which only four progressed to a recto-urethral fistula. Three of the four RUF were unidentified rectal injuries at the time of prostatectomy. Only one of the rectal injuries identified and repaired intraoperatively developed into a RUF. The three patients presenting late required bowel diversion and delayed repair.

Use of radiotherapy for the treatment of prostate cancer has increased dramatically as new techniques are developed and accepted by patients and physicians. External beam radiation therapy (EBRT) was used to treat 20 % of men in the CaPSURE (Cancer of the Prostate Strategic Urological Research Endeavor) database between 1993 and 2001 [4]. The use of brachytherapy increased from 4 % to 22 % during the same time period. Multimodality therapy is also increasing. In those with high-risk features, radiation is frequently recommended following radical prostatectomy in the adjuvant or salvage settings. Additionally, patients with high-risk disease being treated for cure may choose to undergo combined brachytherapy and EBRT. This increased use of XRT has invariably led to increased rates of radiation induced RUF. Contemporary series report that more than 50 % of RUF are caused or complicated by radiation and/or ablation techniques [5, 6]. These risks are magnified further in men undergoing combined external beam and brachytherapy [7]. That being said, RUF formation after radiation therapy remains infrequent, with incidence rates reported from 0 to 0.6 % after EBRT and 0.3–3 % after brachytherapy [5, 8–10].

Radiotherapy may contribute to RUF formation in a variety of ways. Radiation causes both direct and indirect cellular damage through its ionizing effects [11]. Indirect cytotoxicity occurs secondary to the release of oxygen free radicals, altering normal DNA biology and protein synthesis. Direct effects occur when the photon itself damages DNA or tissue proteins. Acute effects of radiation are primarily tissue edema and inflam-

mation with a reduction in cell proliferation. This lack of proliferation may lead to ulceration, bleeding and infection. Subacute and chronic phases are dominated by ischemia and fibrosis. Microvascular damage leads to tissue ischemia, promoting necrosis, fibrosis and worsening ulceration, all of which contribute to radiation induced RUF formation [12]. Effects of radiation are dose and tissue dependent. Higher doses delivered (as with combined brachytherapy and EBRT) will result in higher risk of normal tissue damage and urinary complications. Additionally radiation effects are remarkably tissue dependent. Tissues with high rates of metabolic activity, such as urinary and gastrointestinal epithelium, are most sensitive to the effects of radiation. They are also fixed midline structures that are more difficult to exclude from the radiation fields when treating pelvic malignancies.

The risk of RUF following radiotherapy invariably increases with urethral manipulation, whether endoscopic, open or percutaneous. Men with rectal bleeding following XRT, especially after brachytherapy, should be cautioned against anterior rectal wall biopsy or cautery. This has been shown to induce RUF formation and bleeding usually subsides on its own without intervention [10, 12]. Urinary obstruction is possible after both EBRT and brachytherapy; however, it is more often described with the permanent implant. Rates of obstruction requiring transurethral resection of the prostate (TURP) following brachytherapy range from 0 to 8.3 % [10]. These patients are at high risk for RUF if a complete resection is performed secondary to insufficient blood supply to the prostatic urethra and poor urethral healing [12]. The bladder neck should be spared in these men, if possible, to preserve adequate urethral perfusion. The risks during outlet procedures are not limited to TURP. Experience suggests that RUF formation may be even more likely following prostate laser photovaporization in post-radiation patients. This may be secondary to less control with depth of tissue penetration during laser photovaporization procedures, though RUF rates in this population are not well reported.

PSA recurrence following definitive radiotherapy is not uncommon. CapSURE database analysis found up to 63 % of men developed recurrence a mean 38 months following XRT. In the subset with presumed local recurrence, local salvage treatments may be offered. Salvage radical prostatectomy is most often performed at select high volume centers; however, despite surgeon experience, morbidity with this procedure remains high. Gotto et al. presented a large series of salvage radical prostatectomies and noted a significantly increased risk for RUF compared with primary RP regardless of the type of XRT the patient had previously received [13]. Overall, surgical complications were found in more than 50 % of men.

Cryotherapy is becoming a more commonly performed salvage treatment in the USA secondary to the relative ease of performing the procedure in the salvage setting and the perceived reduced risk of morbidity compared with salvage RP. Although improvements have been made in later generation devices to reduce complications, salvage cryotherapy has been shown to induce RUF formation in 0–3.4 % of men [14]. This risk remains despite performing focal compared to whole gland salvage [15]. Other salvage options following failed EBRT, including brachytherapy and high-intensity focused ultrasound (HIFU), appear to have similar urethrorectal complications. Brachytherapy after EBRT failure leads to RUF formation in an average 3.1 % of men and fistula complications after HIFU approach 4 % [16–18].

Presentation

Iatrogenic rectourethral fistulas secondary to radical prostatectomy typically present within 2–3 weeks following surgery [2, 19]. Radiation induced fistula generally develop in a delayed fashion and typically present between 2 and 3 years following completion of XRT [5, 12]. Clinical symptoms can be variable, though the most commonly reported symptoms are pneumaturia and anal urinary leakage. Those without overt symptoms of a RUF may present with recurrent urinary tract infections and the index of suspicion must be high in those with a history of a radical prostatectomy, especially if a rectal

injury was known to occur during RP. In addition to symptoms commonly found with iatrogenic surgical fistulas, radiation induced fistulas may lead to hematuria, rectal bleeding and pelvic pain. Massive rectal bleeding and necrotizing fasciitis have also been reported with RUF [20].

Fecaluria, a traditional hallmark of urorectal fistulas, is less commonly seen with RUF compared with colovesical fistulas from diverticular disease or malignancy. This is thought to be secondary to the relative high pressure within the urethra compared with the rectum during voiding, leading to rectal urine leakage rather than fecaluria [21]. For this reason, fecaluria is a poor prognostic sign in men with RUF as this would suggest a larger fistula at presentation. It has similarly been suggested that those without fecaluria may be more likely to close spontaneously with urinary diversion with or without colostomy [2].

Diagnosis and Evaluation

An example of a diagnostic and treatment algorithm can be found in Fig. 8.1. Exam under anesthesia allows excellent characterization of the rectourethral fistula and helps with the treatment plan. Digital rectal examination can allow palpation of the fistula if the defect is sufficiently large. Proctoscopy and cystoscopy should both be performed to determine the exact location, size and inflammation associated with the fistula. Fistula tract biopsy should be performed in every patient prior to surgery to rule out recurrent or radiation induced malignancy. Patients should also be evaluated for rectal stenosis as this is found commonly after radiation and may complicate attempts at repair if the stenosis is significant [22].

Retrograde urethrogram (RUG) may be may be performed while the patient is under anesthesia or in the office setting. This will aid in further delineating the location and size of the fistulous tract. If done with the patient awake in the office, concomitant voiding cystourethrogram (VCUG) should also be performed (Fig. 8.2). This will provide additional information with regard to bladder neck and posterior urethral pathology,

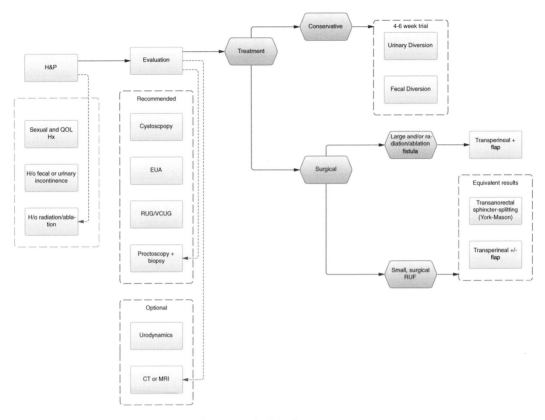

Fig. 8.1 Workup and treatment algorithm for rectourethral fistulas

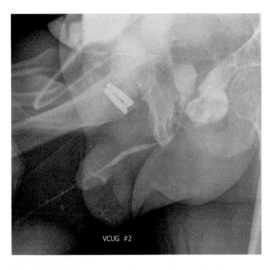

Fig. 8.2 Voiding cystourethrogram demonstrating a rectourethral fistula

such as urethrovesical anastomotic stenosis or prostatic urethral stricture.

Cross sectional abdominopelvic imaging using either computed tomography (CT) or magnetic resonance imaging (MRI) may be indicated in cases where the standard workup is insufficient and the anatomy of the fistula is not clear. This imaging is also helpful in men with prior failed repairs. Some have also suggested that MRI allows demonstration of an intervening cavity between the rectum and urethra, which may aid in surgical planning and patient counseling [21].

Urodynamic testing is occasionally helpful in the evaluation of a rectourethral fistula, though they are often difficult to perform depending on the size of the fistula tract and volume of urine leakage. If they are performed, an assessment of bladder capacity is helpful. Men with radiation induced RUF will frequently also have a reduced bladder capacity. As a consequence, some will be better served with a cystectomy and urinary diversion rather than attempts at fistula repair.

Lastly, men presenting with urorectal fistulas should be evaluated for sexual function and overall quality of life. Erectile function is known to be poor in men with radiation induced RUF [11]. Men considering fistula surgery who have adequate erectile function should be counseled that surgical treatment might result in worsening of their erection quality.

Conservative and Endoscopic Management

Conservative management of rectourethral fistulas generally refers to transurethral or suprapubic urinary drainage in conjunction with a "low residue" diet or temporary colostomy to reduce rectal fecal burden. This regimen is continued for 4–6 weeks and followed by repeat fistula assessment with an office RUG and VCUG. Extending the trial of conservative management beyond 6 weeks for those with a persistent RUF would be futile and those patients should be counseled on surgical options at that time.

Any attempts at conservative management of rectourethral fistulas should reserved for those men with small, surgically induced fistula without associated radiation or tissue ablation injury. This group of patients has the best chance for non-surgical resolution of their fistula. It is likely that rather than a true rectourethral fistula, this situation represents an iatrogenic urorectal communication that has not been present for sufficient time to form an epithelial tract. In this specific scenario, urinary diversion and dietary changes may allow healing to occur before an epithelialized communication becomes permanent.

Several authors have reported positive results using this conservative management technique in surgical RUF. Most recently, Thomas and colleagues reported on 12 patients with a surgically induced fistula who underwent attempts at conservative management with urinary drainage +/− diverting colostomy [2]. Of the 12 men, five (42 %) had resolution of their fistula without surgical intervention. Fecaluria was found to be a negative prognostic sign for fistula resolution with conservative treatment, suggesting that patients with fecaluria have larger and more complex fistulas. Others have also noted some success with conservative measures. Nyam and Pemberton demonstrated at 14 % success rate, and Al-Ali and associates a 46.5 % closure with a similar treatment paradigm [23, 24].

Contrary to an uncomplicated surgical fistula, however, men with a history of radiation or tissue ablation are significantly less likely experience spontaneous closure [5]. These fistulas are complicated by generally being larger in size with inflamed and poorly vascularized surrounding tissue. They also more often present in a delayed fashion when an epithelial tract has had ample time to establish. All of these factors contribute to lack of spontaneous closure.

In addition to urinary and fecal diversion, minimally invasive endoscopic treatments have been attempted for small fistulas. Dolay et al. published a successful case of successful RUF treatment with endoscopic injection of fibrin glue into the fistula tract and rectal mucosal clipping [25]. A similar case report demonstrated success injecting fibrin glue into a complex RUF secondary to rectal Crohn's disease. The fistula resolved and had not recurred at 3 years of follow up [26]. We have also attempted a technique of injecting fibrin glue in men with small and uncomplicated RUF with some success, though small numbers. Fibrin glue theoretically works in these patients by occluding the fistula tract, promoting native fibrin deposition and stimulating fibroblast proliferation. It also stimulates epithelialization and neovascularity, all of which promote fistula resolution. This technique may be an option for those men with uncomplicated fistulas who fail conservative measures and either refuse or are not candidates for a definitive open repair. However, a standardized technique and more robust outcome data are necessary before this minimally invasive treatment option can be broadly recommended.

Open Surgical Management

The vast majority of rectourethral fistulas will require open surgical management. There are several basic surgical principles for optimization of outcomes with fistula repair. No matter which technique is chosen, complete excision of the fistula tract followed by a multilayer, tension free rectal and urethral closure is mandatory. In all but the simplest surgical fistulas, tissue interposition, usually accomplished with a local flap, will improve outcomes. Flaps are especially necessary for any redo procedures or large RUF associated with radiation and/or tissue ablation techniques [6]. Tissue interposition creates a space of separation between the prior fistulous communication and reduces the likelihood of fistula recurrence.

Timing of open repair is often dictated by surgeon preference and experience. It is generally our practice, and that of others, to wait 3 months after a diagnosis surgical fistula with urinary diversion +/− fecal diversion before proceeding with repair [6, 27, 28]. This allows the patient at least an attempt at spontaneous closure and gives time for tissue infection and inflammation to improve or resolve. In men with radiation induced fistulas or RUF following tissue ablation techniques we generally wait 4–6 months as the associated tissue inflammation and tissue necrosis is significantly increased in this group. Men presenting with sepsis or local infection must be adequately treated and fecal diversion is nearly always necessary in this group preoperatively. In those instances we will frequently delay repair slightly longer to allow sufficient tissue healing and resolution of infection.

Preoperative preparation depends on whether the patient has already undergone fecal diversion with a colostomy or ileostomy. If fecal diversion is planned as part of the fistula repair, a full polyethylene glycol mechanical bowel preparation ensures a stool free rectum during surgery. If a fecal diversion was performed prior to fistula repair this is unnecessary. IV antibiotics that cover both skin and gastrointestinal flora are administered within 1 h of incision. Patients with a prior fecal diversion can be fed immediately following surgery. Those undergoing diversion at the time of fistula repair or if electing to undergo repair without a covering fecal diversion should are kept NPO until return of bowel function.

Postoperative care depends on the fistula etiology. Urinary diversion is managed for all patients with a suprapubic tube (SPT) and Foley catheter following RUF repair. The Foley is kept in place for 3–4 weeks and a VCUG is performed at the time of Foley removal confirming the fistula resolution and absence of urethral stricture or bladder neck stenosis. If a fecal diversion is present, this is generally maintained for 3 months following fistula repair. Prior to reversing the diversion, repeat endoscopic and radiographic examination of the urethra is recommended to ensure complete resolution of the fistula tract.

Transanorectal (York Mason and Parks Procedure)

Historically colorectal surgeons rather than urologists performed the majority of rectourethral fistula repairs. As a consequence, surgical approaches utilized for other colorectal surgeries were more commonly used during fistula repair. Although innumerable techniques have been described, transanorectal procedure can broadly be divided into sphincter-splitting approaches (York Mason [29–31]) or more recently the sphincter-preserving transanal rectal advancement flaps (Parks procedure [32]).

Bevan was the first to describe transsphincteric rectal surgery in 1917 for rectal tumors [33]. Its application for the treatment of rectourethral fistulas, however, was not reported until 1969 by Kilpatrick and York Mason [29]. Transanorectal procedures begin by placing the patient in prone jackknife position. The buttocks are spread with adhesive tape. An incision is then made in the midline from the coccyx to the anal verge. The external sphincter is divided with care to place paired sutures at each level of the muscle. These sutures ensure proper sphincter alignment during reconstruction at the completion of the procedure. The rectum is then opened posteriorly along the incision, allowing exposure of the fistula tract. The fistula is sharply excised with a scalpel.

Prospectively catheterizing the fistula tract can be helpful during this portion of the case, but is not mandatory. After the fistula and associated inflammatory tissue has been excised, the rectum and urethra mobilized to allow sufficient separation. A tension free, layered closure of the urethral and rectal defects is then performed with absorbable suture. Three layers of tissue are utilized. The urethra is closed first over a Foley catheter. A substantial layer of anterior rectal wall muscle is approximated second followed by the rectal mucosa, which comprises the third layer. The sphincter is reconstructed and the presacral and overlying tissues cover the defect.

The largest experience with the transanorectal modified York Mason approach to RUF repair was presented in 2012 by Hadley and colleagues from the University of Utah [34]. Fifty one patients at their institution underwent this approach to fistula repair over their 40 year experience. Only seven patients had radiation-induced fistulas with the remainder surgical fistulas. To date they have only experience five fistula recurrences with a greater than 90 % success rate. One of the failures was salvaged with a repeat York Mason procedure. The remainder underwent permanent urinary or fecal diversion. A summary of outcomes from this and other select series using this technique can be found in Table 8.1.

The other less commonly used transanal technique for RUF repair is a sphincter-sparing rectal advancement flap, or Parks procedure [32]. This approach is also performed in the prone jackknife position and involves transanal fistula exposure without incising the rectal sphincter or mucosa. Exposure is achieved with fixed anal retractors. Once the tract has been identified, a U-shaped broad based flap of rectal mucosa and muscle is raised. The apex of the U is situated through the fistula tract and the tract is excised. The defect is then closed in three layers: urethral mucosa approximated over the Foley catheter, rectal wall/muscle and rectal mucosa.

The rectal advancement technique is less commonly used, even by colorectal surgeons, secondary to reduced exposure and difficulty with fistula excision and repair. Garofalo et al. published a 20-year experience with rectal advancement flaps for RUF repair [35]. Over that time period only 12 men underwent attempts at fistula treatment utilizing this technique. At a mean follow up of 31 months, eight patients (67 %) were free from RUF recurrence. More recently, Joshi and associates presented their results with five patients using this technique [36]. All five men are asymptomatic without fistula recurrence at a median 11 months, though one did require a second procedure after failure of the initial attempt (80 % success at first attempt).

Although initially the mainstay of rectourethral fistula surgery, sphincter-splitting and preserving transanal fistula repairs are now much less frequently utilized. Sphincter preserving procedures are only useful in those men with small, distal, non-irradiated RUF in whom a more minimally invasive approach seems optimal. This approach is severely limited in its exposure and has no place in the treatment of larger fistula or those with associated radiation or tissue ablation injury. Additionally, while the urethra may be closed using this technique, rectal flap advancement is the primary means for fistula resolution. This ignores the presumption that the pressure gradient favors flow from the urethra into the rectum rather than vice versa [21]. That being said, morbidity following a transanal procedure is low and it does not preclude a transperineal salvage should the initial attempt at closure fail.

Sphincter-splitting transanal approaches are performed more commonly than sphincter-preserving ones and have demonstrated comparable outcomes to transperineal repairs (88 % overall operative success) [42]. However, this approach is limited in its versatility. Treatment of concomitant bladder neck stenosis or urethral stricture is not possible with a transrectal approach and interposition flaps can be more difficult. Ideal candidates are those with small-moderate sized fistulas (<2 cm) without a history of prior radiotherapy or tissue ablation. Men with larger fistulas or those with other complicating factors who undergo a transrectal repair are known to be at a significant disadvantage, demonstrating reduced operative success compared to small, non-radiated fistulas [34].

Table 8.1 Select large rectourethral fistula series and outcomes [5, 6, 23, 24, 28, 34–41]

Study	Year	Total RUF patients	H/o XRT or tissue ablation, n (%)	Temporary fecal diversion, n (%)	Resolution with conservative treatment, n (%)	Transanal, sphincter sparing, n (%)	Transanorectal, sphincter-splitting, n (%)	Transabdominal, n (%)	Transperineal, n (%)	Tissue flap usage Any, n (%)	Gracilis, n	Omentum, n	Other, n	Successful surgical RUF closure, n (%)	Mean follow up, months
Hadley et al.	2012	51	8 (16)	20 (39)	–	–	51 (100)	–	–	2 (6)	2	–	–	46/51 (90)	NR
Garofalo et al.	2003	23	3 (13)	16 (70)	4 (17)	14 (61)	3 (13)	2 (9)	–	–	–	–	–	13/19 (68)	31 ± 33.4
Joshi et al.	2011	5	–	3 (60)	–	5 (100)	–	–	–	–	–	–	–	4 (80)	11 (4–24)
Al-Ali et al.	1997	30	–	30 (100)	14 (47)	1 (3)	11 (37)	3 (10)	1 (3)	2 (12.5)	–	2	–	14/16 (87.5)	66 (18–132)
Rouanne et al.	2011	10	–	10 (100)	–	–	10 (100)	–	–	–	–	–	–	10/10 (100)	24 (18–28)
Kasraeian et al.	2009	12	2 (17)	6 (50)	–	–	12 (100)	–	–	–	–	–	–	9/12 (75)	22 (2–73)
Vanni et al.	2010	74	39 (53)	73 (98.6)	–	–	–	–	74 (100)	74 (100)	68	–	6	68/74 (92)	20
Voelzke et al.	2013	23	13 (57)	21 (91)	–	–	–	–	23 (100)	7 (30)	2	–	5	18/23 (78)	13 (3–39)
Ulrich et al.	2009	26	14 (54)	26 (100)	–	–	–	–	26 (100)	26 (100)	26	–	–	26 (100)	22 ± 14
Ghoniem et al.	2008	25	17 (68)	25 (100)	–	–	–	–	25 (100)	25 (100)	25	–	–	25 (100)	28 (3–132)
Wexner et al.	2008	36	20 (56)	36 (100)	–	–	–	–	36 (100)	36 (100)	36	–	–	28 (78)	NR
Lane et al.	2006	22	22 (100)	20 (91)	5 (23)	–	1 (4.5)	15 (68)	1 (4.5)	4 (24)	2	2	–	15/17 (88)	29
Nyam et al.	1999	16	7 (44)	7 (44)	3 (18.75)	2 (12.5)	2 (12.5)	3 (18.75)	6 (37.5)	3 (23)	NR	NR	NR	9/13 (69)	80 (8–180)

In the last 15–20 years, the proportion of men presenting with symptoms of a RUF who have previously been radiated has increased dramatically. Prior to 1997, 4 % of RUF were complicated by radiation whereas more than 50 % present with that history today [5, 6]. Thus, finding an ideal patient for a transanorectal procedure is becoming increasingly difficult. Additionally, although it has not been reported in the literature, concern for anal incontinence with a sphincter-splitting procedure is pervasive, especially with surgeons less familiar with this approach. For these reasons, some have argued that a transperineal approach to fistula repair is more adaptable to any situation and should be the procedure of choice for both uncomplicated and complicated fistulas [21].

Transperineal

A perineal approach to repair of rectourethral fistulas is becoming increasingly common and now represents the preferred technique for RUF surgery. Perineal exposure is something most urologists are comfortable with, given its use in a variety of urologic surgeries, including urethroplasty, incontinence procedures, urethrectomy, and others. In addition to addressing the RUF, this technique allows the treatment of concomitant bladder neck and urethral pathology in the same setting and is ideally situated for raising local flaps for tissue interposition.

The perineal approach to RUF repair begins with the patient in dorsal lithotomy or exaggerated lithotomy position. We most often utilized exaggerated lithotomy as this allows two surgeons to comfortably operate standing side-by-side, but this is a matter of surgeon preference. An inverted "U" or lambda incision is made in the perineum. The Jordan-Simpson perineal Bookwalter retractor or similar perineal retractor is helpful for exposure. The transverse perinei muscles are divided and the perineal body is completely incised. This allows the urethra to be elevated and a surgical plane developed in close proximity to the anterior rectum all the way up to the peritoneum. The rectum and ure-thra are widely mobilized and the fistula is divided and exposed.

Closure of both the rectum and urethra depend on the size of the fistula and resulting tissue defect. The rectum should always be closed in horizontal layers to avoid iatrogenic rectal stenosis. Larger fistulas may require more thorough rectal mobilization to close tension free, whereas smaller fistulas require less mobility. Small urethral defects are easily approximated over a Foley catheter in two layers. If the fistula is sufficiently large such that a primary closure is not possible, a tissue interposition is required. We prefer a buccal mucosa graft (BMG) onlay in this scenario, which allows closure of nearly any size urethral defect. When using a BMG, a vascularized bed is necessary to support the graft [43]. Depending on the location of the graft, this is most often accomplished with a gracilis muscle flap, but ischiocavernosus muscle, Singapore flap, levator muscle, or other healthy local tissue flap may be used. In addition to reducing the chance for recurrent RUF, the flap functions to fill the cavity with healthy tissue to promote imbibition and inosculation of the graft.

A significant advantage of the perineal approach is its versatility for men with concomitant urethral strictures or urethrovesical anastomotic stenosis. Urethral strictures can be approached in the same fashion as a primary urethroplasty with a few important distinctions. We generally favor non-transecting techniques for repair of urethral strictures in this setting to preserve urethral vascularity and promote healing. The proximal bulbourethral blood supply is often, if not always, sacrificed or damaged prior to or during fistula repair. For this reason, retrograde distal arterial supply from the dorsal and cavernosal arteries is exquisitely important. Bulbomembranous strictures can be managed with a ventral urethrotomy, extending the fistula tract through the strictured region. A longer BMG is then placed ventrally with a gracilis muscle flap for support. For strictures distant from the site of the fistula this technique is not feasible and we favor urethral mobilization and a dorsal urethrotomy and BMG onlay technique. Men with concomitant urethrovesical anastomotic stenosis may be managed with urethral mobilization, excision of the stricture segment and complete revision of the urethrovesical anastomosis. An inferior pubectomy may be required in these patients for adequate visualization of the bladder neck for repair. Alternatively an abdominaoperineal approach may be chosen, but we have not found this necessary in the majority of cases.

The largest series of transperineal RUF surgery was published by Vanni et al. in 2010 [6]. They retrospectively reported on 74 patients who underwent RUF repair at their institution. Of the 74 patients, 35 were non-radiated surgical RUF and 39 were radiation induced fistulas. An interposition flap was used in all patients, including a gracilis muscle flap in 92 % and a range of other flaps in the remainder. Urethral strictures were concurrently treated with BMG onlay in 11 % and 28 % of men in the radiated and non-radiated groups, respectively. At a mean follow up of 20 months, 100 % of the non-radiated men and 84 % of the radiated men were free of fistula recurrence in a single stage. Thirty-one percent of radiated patients required permanent fecal diversion secondary to permanent rectal damage or a noncompliant anal sphincter.

Several other centers have published results with transperineal repair of RUF (Table 8.1). Mundy and Andrich reported on 40 patients utilizing this technique (23 surgical, 17 radiation fistulas) [21]. A purely perineal approach was used in all surgical fistulas, however for radiation induced fistulas an abdominoperineal approach was performed in 14 of the 17 men. This allowed the fistula surgery to be combined with a salvage radical prostatectomy in eight men. With a minimal of 1 year follow up on each patient, 100 % of patient had resolution of their fistula, though some did require prolonged catheter drainage before complete healing of the urethra on urethrography.

More recently, Voelzke and associates reviewed their outcomes with a perineal approach to RUF repair in 23 patients. Different from the dorsal lithotomy position used in most perineal surgery, they opted for a prone jackknife position

in 15 of the 23 men. Their rationale for this technique alteration was to reduce the exposure limitations, which are inevitable with the anterior pubic arch. As with transsphincteric procedures, however, this position limits ability to easily perform a gracilis muscle interposition flap. In this series a flap was utilized in only 7 of the 23 patients. At a mean 13 months of follow up, they found 100 % success rate in the surgical fistulas and 61.5 % with the radiation/ablation fistulas.

Transperineal approaches to RUF repair have many advantages over transrectal, sphincter-preserving or splitting procedures. This technique allows concurrent treatment of both urethral strictures and bladder neck contractures, both of which are found commonly in RUF patients, especially those with a history of radiation. Recent publications report a 25–30 % risk for concomitant bulbomembranous or bladder neck strictures in men with a radiation induced RUF [6, 28]. With patients already in the appropriate position for repair of that pathology it can be performed in the same setting without need for unnecessary repeat surgery through a complicated surgical field. The perineal approach is also the easiest with which to perform tissue interposition flaps, specifically the gracilis flap that is most commonly used. While it is possible to use a gracilis flap in the prone position, this may require harvesting the flap ahead of time with subsequent patient repositioning, adding time and potential complications to an already difficult procedure [28]. Finally, a perineal approach in the lithotomy position offers the opportunity to easily progress to an abdominoperineal procedure if a salvage prostatectomy or other concurrent procedures are necessary.

Gracilis Muscle Flap

The need for tissue interposition during RUF surgery is debated. Some high-volume centers argue that in uncomplicated small surgical fistulas a flap is unnecessary [21, 28]. Others suggest that flaps offer an important protection against fistula recurrence, even in a patient with a straightforward RUF [6]. Most would agree, however, that for radiation or ablation induced fistulas, tissue interposition reduces the risk for recurrence and is strongly recommended.

The gracilis muscle peninsular flap for use in rectourethral fistula repair was initially described by Ryan et al. in 1979 [44]. Since the initial description it has been widely accepted and now represents the most common flap used during RUF surgery. It has been consistently proven to offer excellent outcomes compared with other local tissue flaps [6, 27, 37, 38]. While no randomized trials exist, small comparative studies do show an advantage with the addition of a gracilis flap interposition compared with no flap for RUF repairs [23]. A primary reason for widespread acceptance of this flap for perineal surgery is its versatility. It can be harvested from one or both legs without significant morbidity or loss of function. It is consistently present in patients regardless of age or gender, and it easily rotates into the perineum without tension. Finally, the proximal pedicle off the profunda femoris is hardy and flap necrosis is rare as long as an adequate tunnel is created.

The gracilis muscle is a long (25–30 cm), thin muscle originating at the ischiopubic ramus and inserting on the medial condyle of the tibia (Table 8.2). The predominant vascular pedicle is supplied by the medial circumflex femoral artery, which is a branch of the profunda femoris on the proximal aspect. The pedicle can usually be found about 10 cm from the gracilis muscle origin. Distal pedicles are small branches off the superficial femoral artery and can be sacrificed without concern for flap compromise. One or two

vessels comprise the primary venous drainage and usually accompany the artery.

With the patient in lithotomy position, the muscle belly can be palpated between two fingers at the medial thigh approximately 10 cm from the ischiopubic ramus, marking the approximate point of the primary vascular pedicle (Fig. 8.3a). A medial thigh incision is made from this point distally towards the site of insertion. The incision can either be extended all the way to the tendinous insertion or alternatively a counter-incision can be made at that point. The dominant vascular pedicle is prospectively identified early, such that distal dissection can proceed quickly. A vascular Doppler can be used to aid in locating the vessel if it is difficult. Once the artery has been safely marked the muscle is circumferentially controlled with a Penrose drain for retraction (Fig. 8.3b, c). The distal attachments can be bluntly freed with selective use of electrocautery. With the muscle mobilized to its insertion, the proper tendinous attachment is confirmed with gentle traction on the muscle while palpating the tendon. It can then be incised with cautery. The gracilis muscle is then rotated back 180° through the thigh incision towards the perineum (Fig. 8.3d). Care must be taken not to twist the flap and occlude the arterial supply. A generous subcutaneous tunnel is created from the thigh incision into the perineal incision; the muscle is transposed and sutured in place (Fig. 8.3e). The thigh is closed in layers and a closed suction drain is left for several days. A compressive wrap on the leg may be placed to reduce the risk for hematoma formation.

Though not well documented in the literature, complications following gracilis muscle harvest appear to be minimal and the procedure well tolerated. The gracilis muscle functions to medially rotate and adduct the hip as well as flex the knee. After the muscle is harvested the adductor longus and magnus replace the functionality and motor defects have not been reported [38]. There is a small risk for hematoma formation with gracilis harvest, especially if a minimal incision is attempted with counter-incision over the insertion site. This requires

Table 8.2 Gracilis muscle characteristics

Function	Medial hip rotation and adduction, knee flexion
Size	4–8 cm width; 25–30 cm length (depending on leg size)
Arterial supply	Medial circumflex femoral artery (branch of profunda femoris)
Origin	Ischiopubic ramus
Insertion	Medial tibial condyle

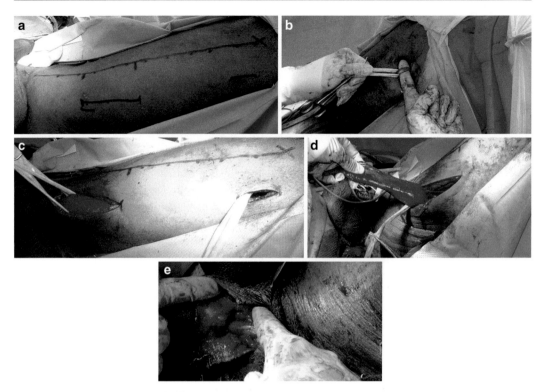

Fig. 8.3 (**a–e**) Intraoperative photos during gracilis flap harvesting. Preoperative skin marking demonstrate the approximate location for the dominant vascular pedicle (**a**). A skin incision overlying the muscle belly allows dis- section of the muscle with a counter incision for transec- tion of the tendon (**b, c**). The muscle is rotated 180° (**d**), tunneled and sutured in place in the perineum (**e**)

blind dissection and vessels may not be ade- quately controlled. The postoperative compres- sive wrap should help to reduce this risk.

Minimally Invasive Surgical Management

Minimally invasive approaches to rectourethral fistulas are in their infancy and have been described only in case reports and small series of three to four patients. Sotelo and colleagues published their results with two patients perform- ing a purely laparoscopic fistula repair [45]. One patient developed a fistula after a low anterior resection for rectal cancer and was managed with a simple laparoscopic prostatectomy and fistula closure. The neurovascular bundles were used for tissue interposition. Another patient developed a RUF after radical prostatectomy with the fistula

near the urethrovesical anastomosis. This fistula was managed with a laparoscopic, transvesical approach. The tract was excised, rectum closed and an omental flap was interposed. No fistula recurrences were reported.

Gozen and colleagues have also reported on two patients undergoing laparoscopic RUF repair. In both cases, a laparoscopic prostatec- tomy was performed followed by rectal closure and urethrovesical anastomosis. A peritoneal flap was used in one patient and a tunica vaginalis flap in another for interposition. No recurrences were noted at more than 8 months follow up.

Laparoscopic surgery is now widely accepted for many urologic procedures. Its use in rectoure- thral fistula repair, however, is only beginning to be described. While a technique utilizing robotic assistance has never been published, this technol- ogy certainly has the potential to make a laparo- scopic fistula repair less daunting. However, the merits of a minimally invasive approach to RUF repair has not, and may never be, adequately articulated. Morbidity associated with either transperineal or transrectal fistula surgery is minimal, the risk for postoperative ileus is low, and there is no risk for damage to intra-abdominal structures. None of these can be stated confidently with laparoscopic approaches for fistula closure. Experienced laparoscopic surgeons must describe consistent results and a reliable technique before it can be accepted as an option in the fistula armamentarium.

Conclusions

Rectourethral fistulas today are most often a rare complication from the treatment of prostate cancer. When they do occur, however, patients suffer significant morbidity with negative effects on quality of life. Contemporary large series of RUF report a dramatic increase in the complexity of men presenting with RUF. While most RUF were formerly surgical fistulas without associated radiation injury, patients with RUF presenting today are frequently caused by or complicated by a history of radiation and tissue ablation techniques. Unfortunately, these complex fistulas are often larger, more difficult to treat, and have proven to have worse outcomes following surgical correction compared with uncomplicated RUF. Liberal use of tissue interposition flaps, such as the gracilis muscle flap, as well as judicious application of fecal diversion will optimize patient outcomes. While the vast majority of patients can be successfully cured, men with end-stage bladders and large complex fistulas may be best managed with cystectomy and urinary diversion and should be counseled on that option.

References

1. Bukowski TP, Chakrabarty A, Powell IJ, et al. Acquired rectourethral fistula: methods of repair. J Urol. 1995;153:730–3.
2. Thomas C, Jones J, Jager W, et al. Incidence, clinical symptoms and management of rectourethral fistulas after radical prostatectomy. J Urol. 2010;183:608–12.
3. Wedmid A, Mendoza P, Sharma S, et al. Rectal injury during robot-assisted radical prostatectomy: incidence and management. J Urol. 2011;186:1928–33.
4. Cooperberg MR, Broering JM, Litwin MS, et al. The contemporary management of prostate cancer in the United States: lessons from the cancer of the prostate strategic urologic research endeavor (CapSURE), a national disease registry. J Urol. 2004;171:1393–401.
5. Lane BR, Stein DE, Remzi FH, et al. Management of radiotherapy induced rectourethral fistula. J Urol. 2006;175:1382–7. discussion 1387-8, 2006.
6. Vanni AJ, Buckley JC, Zinman LN. Management of surgical and radiation induced rectourethral fistulas with an interposition muscle flap and selective buccal mucosal onlay graft. J Urol. 2010;184:2400–4.
7. Marguet C, Raj GV, Brashears JH, et al. Rectourethral fistula after combination radiotherapy for prostate cancer. Urology. 2007;69:898–901.
8. Pisansky TM, Kozelsky TF, Myers RP, et al. Radiotherapy for isolated serum prostate specific antigen elevation after prostatectomy for prostate cancer. J Urol. 2000;163:845 50.
9. Theodorescu D, Gillenwater JY, Koutrouvelis PG. Prostatourethral-rectal fistula after prostate brachytherapy. Cancer. 2000;89:2085–91.
10. Stone NN, Stock RG. Complications following permanent prostate brachytherapy. Eur Urol. 2002;41:427–33.
11. Ballek NK, Gonzalez CM. Reconstruction of radiation-induced injuries of the lower urinary tract. Urol Clin North Am. 2013;40:407–19.
12. Chrouser KL, Leibovich BC, Sweat SD, et al. Urinary fistulas following external radiation or permanent brachytherapy for the treatment of prostate cancer. J Urol. 2005;173:1953–7.
13. Gotto GT, Yunis LH, Vora K, et al. Impact of prior prostate radiation on complications after radical prostatectomy. J Urol. 2010;184:136–42.
14. Mouraviev V, Spiess PE, Jones JS. Salvage cryoablation for locally recurrent prostate cancer following primary radiotherapy. Eur Urol. 2012;61:1204–11.
15. Li YH, Elshafei A, Agarwal G et al. Salvage focal prostate cryoablation for locally recurrent prostate cancer after radiotherapy: Initial results from the cryo on-line data registry. Prostate, 2014.
16. Uchida T, Shoji S, Nakano M, et al. High-intensity focused ultrasound as salvage therapy for patients with recurrent prostate cancer after external beam radiation, brachytherapy or proton therapy. BJU Int. 2011;107:378–82.
17. Parekh A, Graham PL, Nguyen PL. Cancer control and complications of salvage local therapy after failure of radiotherapy for prostate cancer: a systematic review. Semin Radiat Oncol. 2013;23:222–34.
18. Netsch C, Bach T, Gross E, et al. Rectourethral fistula after high-intensity focused ultrasound therapy for prostate cancer and its surgical management. Urology. 2011;77:999–1004.
19. Dal Moro F, Mancini M, Pinto F, et al. Successful repair of iatrogenic rectourinary fistulas using the pos-

terior sagittal transrectal approach (York-Mason): 15-year experience. World J Surg. 2006;30:107–13.

20. Cherr GS, Hall C, Pineau BC, et al. Rectourethral fistula and massive rectal bleeding from iodine-125 prostate brachytherapy: a case report. Am Surg. 2001;67:131–4.

21. Mundy AR, Andrich DE. Urorectal fistulae following the treatment of prostate cancer. BJU Int. 2011;107: 1298–303.

22. Turina M, Mulhall AM, Mahid SS, et al. Frequency and surgical management of chronic complications related to pelvic radiation. Arch Surg. 2008;143:46–52. discussion 52, 2008.

23. Nyam DC, Pemberton JH. Management of iatrogenic rectourethral fistula. Dis Colon Rectum. 1999;42:994–7. discussion 997-9, 1999.

24. Al-Ali M, Kashmoula D, Saoud IJ. Experience with 30 posttraumatic rectourethral fistulas: presentation of posterior transsphincteric anterior rectal wall advancement. J Urol. 1997;158:421–4.

25. Dolay K, Aras B, Tugcu V, et al. Combined treatment of iatrogenic rectourethral fistula with endoscopic fibrin glue application and clipping. J Endourol. 2007;21:433–6.

26. Etienney I, Rabahi N, Cuenod CA, et al. Fibrin glue sealing in the treatment of a recto-urethral fistula in Crohn's disease: a case report. Gastroenterol Clin Biol. 2009;33:1094–7.

27. Gupta G, Kumar S, Kekre NS, et al. Surgical management of rectourethral fistula. Urology. 2008;71:267–71.

28. Voelzke BB, McAninch JW, Breyer BN, et al. Transperineal management for postoperative and radiation rectourethral fistulas. J Urol. 2013;189: 966–71.

29. Kilpatrick FR, Mason AY. Post-operative recto-prostatic fistula. Br J Urol. 1969;41:649–54.

30. Prasad ML, Nelson R, Hambrick E, et al. York Mason procedure for repair of postoperative rectoprostatic urethral fistula. Dis Colon Rectum. 1983;26:716–20.

31. Fengler SA, Abcarian H. The York Mason approach to repair of iatrogenic rectourinary fistulae. Am J Surg. 1997;173:213–7.

32. Parks AG, Motson RW. Peranal repair of rectoprostatic fistula. Br J Surg. 1983;70:725–6.

33. Bevan AD. Carcinoma of the rectum: treatment by local excision. Surg Clin Chicago. 1917;1:1233.

34. Hadley DA, Southwick A, Middleton RG. York-Mason procedure for repair of recto-urinary fistulae: a 40-year experience. BJU Int. 2012;109:1095–8.

35. Garofalo TE, Delaney CP, Jones SM, et al. Rectal advancement flap repair of rectourethral fistula: a 20-year experience. Dis Colon Rectum. 2003;46: 762–9.

36. Joshi HM, Vimalachandran D, Heath RM, et al. Management of iatrogenic recto-urethral fistula by transanal rectal flap advancement. Colorectal Dis. 2011;13:918–20.

37. Ghoniem G, Elmissiry M, Weiss E, et al. Transperineal repair of complex rectourethral fistula using gracilis muscle flap interposition—can urinary and bowel functions be preserved? J Urol. 2008;179:1882–6.

38. Ulrich D, Roos J, Jakse G, et al. Gracilis muscle interposition for the treatment of recto-urethral and recto-vaginal fistulas: a retrospective analysis of 35 cases. J Plast Reconstr Aesthet Surg. 2009;62:352–6.

39. Kasraeian A, Rozet F, Cathelineau X, et al. Modified York-Mason technique for repair of iatrogenic rec-tourinary fistula: the Montsouris experience. J Urol. 2009;181:1178–83.

40. Rouanne M, Vaessen C, Bitker MO, et al. Outcome of a modified York Mason technique in men with iatrogenic urethrorectal fistula after radical prostatectomy. Dis Colon Rectum. 2011;54:1008–13.

41. Wexner SD, Ruiz DE, Genua J, et al. Gracilis muscle interposition for the treatment of rectourethral, recto-vaginal, and pouch-vaginal fistulas: results in 53 patients. Ann Surg. 2008;248:39–43.

42. Hechenbleikner EM, Buckley JC, Wick EC. Acquired rectourethral fistulas in adults: a systematic review of surgical repair techniques and outcomes. Dis Colon Rectum. 2013;56:374–83.

43. Zinman L. Muscular, myocutaneous, and fasciocutaneous flaps in complex urethral reconstruction. Urol Clin North Am. 2002;29:443–66. viii.

44. Ryan Jr JA, Beebe HG, Gibbons RP. Gracilis muscle flap for closure of rectourethral fistula. J Urol. 1979; 122:124–5.

45. Sotelo R, Mirandolino M, Trujillo G, et al. Laparoscopic repair of rectourethral fistulas after prostate surgery. Urology. 2007;70:515–8.

Reoperative Anti-incontinence Surgery

9

Brian J. Linder and Daniel S. Elliott

Introduction

Primary surgical management of men with persistent stress urinary incontinence (SUI) following definitive prostate cancer management, either with urethral sling placement or artificial urinary sphincter (AUS) placement, is typically highly successful [1, 2]. However, with either management option, patients may experience persistent or recurrent incontinence. A thorough evaluation of these patients is needed, as there is a broad range of potentially contributing etiologies. Additionally, given the technical considerations inherent to reoperative surgery, including altered anatomy and potentially impaired tissue health, repeat anti-incontinence surgery presents a challenging clinical entity. Here in, we present our approach to management of the most common scenarios for repeat anti-incontinence surgery.

Evaluation of Persistent or Recurrent Urinary Incontinence Following Anti-incontinence Surgery

Evaluation of persistent or recurrent stress urinary incontinence following anti-incontinence surgery requires careful consideration of various potential contributing factors and a stepwise approach to diagnosis. The workup for this issue varies based on the patient's etiology for incontinence, comorbidities, initial anti-incontinence procedure performed and the known risk factors for surgical failure.

With regard to artificial urinary sphincter placement, persistent/recurrent stress incontinence can broadly be categorized into: improper device utilization, mechanical and non-mechanical failures, or non-device related causes. The evaluation of post-AUS incontinence begins with a thorough history, including timing and acuity of onset, concomitant lower urinary tract symptoms such as urinary urgency or frequency, dysuria, hematuria, or urinary tract infections, as well as a focused physical exam. As part of this exam, providers should evaluate the patient's functional knowledge and ability to properly utilize the device. If improper technique is encountered, patients may need reinstruction regarding device function. Additionally, non-device related causes, such as urinary tract infection and overflow incontinence (from decreased bladder

B.J. Linder, M.D. • D.S. Elliott, M.D. (✉)
Department of Urology, Mayo Clinic, 200 First St.
SW, Rochester, MN 55905, USA
e-mail: Elliott.Daniel@mayo.edu

© Springer International Publishing Switzerland 2016
J.S. Sandhu (ed.), *Urinary Dysfunction in Prostate Cancer*, DOI 10.1007/978-3-319-23817-3_9

contractility, urethral stricture or bladder neck contracture) should be assessed for with a urinalysis/urine culture and post-void residual. Likewise, if de novo urinary urgency and urge incontinence are identified in the setting of an otherwise normal evaluation, including cystoscopy, they may be managed with behavioral modification and pharmacotherapy [3].

In the event the above tests are within normal limits, further evaluation is centered on delineating mechanical versus non-mechanical failures.

Mechanical failure is typically determined by evaluating the presence/absence of fluid present in the AUS device, as fluid leakage may lead to inadequate pressure for mucosal copatation. Depending on the fluid utilized during device implantation, normal saline versus dilute contrast, imaging with ultrasound or abdominal X-ray can be performed [4, 5]. We prefer the use of dilute contrast to fill the device as this allows for straightforward in-office evaluation of a potential mechanical failure, as shown in Fig. 9.1.

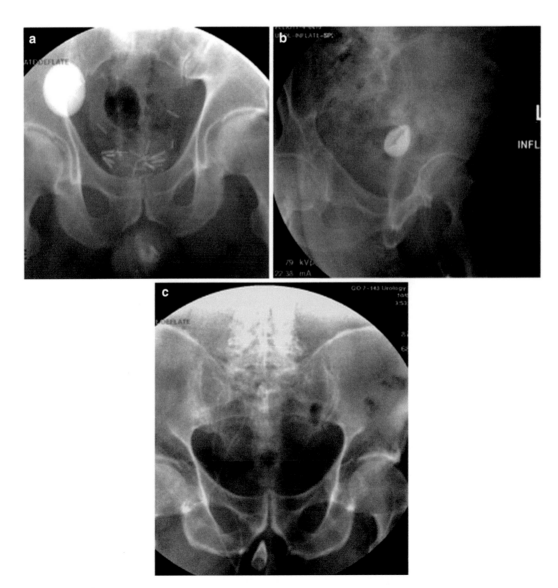

Fig. 9.1 Representative images in the evaluation of mechanical failure. These demonstrate: normal reservoir contour (**a**), early mechanical failure with deformation of the abdominal reservoir (**b**), late mechanical failure with loss of all contrast from the abdominal reservoir (**c**)

It should be noted that without a baseline film for comparison, roughly 50 % of the contrast would need to be extravasated from the abdominal reservoir before changes in the reservoir contour may be detected on plain X-ray [4]. One benefit to filling the system with contrast is that an immediate postoperative X-ray allows for prompt recognition inadequate device filling or issues with connectors.

By comparison, non-mechanical failure, such as improper cuff sizing, urethral atrophy or erosion, is further evaluated with office cystoscopy, including device cycling/manipulation. Overall, urethral atrophy is the most common cause for revision surgery of AUS devices [6, 7]. Urethral atrophy is diagnosed when there is adequate fluid in the system, yet incomplete mucosal coaptation with device cycling during cystoscopy (Fig. 9.2). Likewise, ischemic changes of the urethral tissue underlying the cuff, such as tissue blanching, may be identified. During cystoscopic evaluation for urethral atrophy it important to note the posi-

tion of the current urethral cuff and health of the surrounding urethral tissues as this may impact surgical planning. Similar to urethral atrophy, cystoscopic examination may identify urethral erosion, with visualization of the urethral cuff (Fig. 9.3).

In addition to consideration of the above factors, evaluation of recurrent/persistent incontinence following male urethral sling placement includes further evaluation of sling and bladder function. For instance, sling migration/slippage, from lack of fixation or suture failure, may lead to recurrent/persistent incontinence. This can be evaluated with a repositioning test during office cystoscopy, which may help guide further management [8, 9]. Additionally, if not appreciated preoperatively, impaired bladder compliance or detrusor underactivity may also predispose to sling failure [8]. Thus, consideration can be given to performing a urodynamic evaluation if incontinence persists/recurs after urethral sling placement.

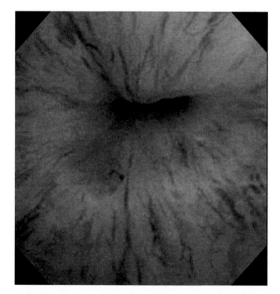

Fig. 9.2 Cystoscopy demonstrating incomplete urethral mucosal coaptation secondary to urethral atrophy

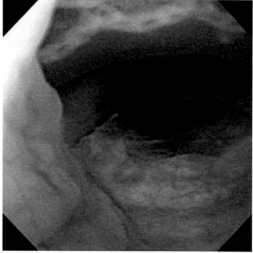

Fig. 9.3 Cystoscopy demonstrating a 180° dorsal urethral erosion

Anti-incontinence Surgery Following a Failed Artificial Urinary Sphincter

While the AUS is the gold standard for surgical management of severe male stress urinary incontinence, with 5 and 10-year device survival rates of roughly 75 % and 65 %, it is prone to failure over time [1, 7, 10, 11]. Of note, understanding the underlying cause of failure is crucial to optimal patient management. Here, we will focus on specific causes for recurrent or persistent SUI following AUS placement and their surgical management. Notably, the mainstay of surgical therapy following a failed AUS, is a repeat AUS as there is limited evidence regarding the efficacy of urethral sling placement in this setting [12, 13]. This is thought to be secondary to periurethral scarring following AUS placement which decreases the ability of the urethral sling to achieve adequate coaptation [12, 14].

Urethral Atrophy

The AUS achieves urinary continence by applying circumferential compression of the spongy tissues surrounding the urethra. While this mechanism of action allows for excellent functional outcomes, even in cases of severe leakage, this chronic pressure can compromise the underlying urethral tissue health and lead to urethral atrophy. In fact, urethral atrophy is the most common cause for a non-mechanical failure or device revision [6, 7, 15]. Typically, patients with urethral atrophy will report a gradual recurrence of stress urinary incontinence. The diagnosis is confirmed during cystoscopy, where incomplete urethral coaptation is visualized with device cycling (with adequate fluid in the system).

The treatment of AUS failure secondary to urethral atrophy is centered on device revision, though other strategies have been reported. Surgical options for AUS revision in cases of urethral atrophy include changing the location of the urethral cuff (moving proximally or distally), downsizing the urethral cuff, placement of a tandem urethral cuff or revising the pressure-regulating balloon. The decision between these management options is

based on the local tissue quality, location of the in situ urethral cuff and surgeon preference.

Initial management of submucosal urethral atrophy is typically with downsizing the urethral cuff [15–17]. An advantage to urethral cuff downsizing is that no additional periurethral dissection is necessary. Of note, while previously downsizing could only occur to a urethral cuff size of 4.0, more recently the 3.5 cm urethral cuff has been introduced. Early reports with this smaller cuff size have been encouraging, though long-term data is lacking [18]. Additionally, an increased rate of erosion has been reported in patients treated with this smaller cuff in the setting of prior pelvic radiation, compared to those without this exposure (21 % versus 4 %) [19].

In cases where the smallest available cuff is already in situ or cuff downsizing has previously failed, other options include: relocation of the urethral cuff, placement of tandem urethral cuffs, or manipulation of the pressure-regulating balloon. Changing the location of the urethral cuff is an excellent option when an area of healthy urethra can be identified in a more proximal or slightly more distal location that would allow for adequate tissue coaptation. Of note, as the caliber of the urethra tapers distally, careful attention must be given to appropriate cuff sizing in order to avoid persistent SUI. In order to account for urethral tapering distally, use of a transcorporal technique for added tissue bulk in the setting of revision for urethral atrophy has been described [20].

Another management strategy for submucosal urethral atrophy is placement of a tandem urethral cuff. Tandem urethral cuff placement attempts to avoid increasing the pressure on the atrophic urethra segment and instead distributes additional compression to a second area of the urethra [21]. With regard to the technique of tandem urethral cuff placement, circumferential urethral dissection roughly 2 cm distal to the primary cuff is needed (Fig. 9.4a). In cases with difficult tissue planes, a transcorporal approach to tandem cuff placement can be utilized [22]. The device tubing emanating from the existing cuff is dissected free, controlled with rubber shods and transected. Following this the new cuff is attached with the use of a Y-shaped adapter and Prolene free-ties (Fig. 9.4b). We prefer to use this approach, rather than additional Quick-Connect attachments in the perineum, as these are more bulky and have in some cases have led to cutaneous erosions. Notably, given the additional urethral cuff, we typically add 3 cc of fluid (normal saline or contrast) to the system. Notably, excellent surgical outcomes have been reported with a tandem cuff technique [21, 23]. However, compared to single cuff placement, tandem cuff placement may have higher rate of urinary retention and revision surgery [24]. Additionally, higher rates of erosion have been associated with distal urethral cuff placement [25].

An additional option for AUS revision for recurrent incontinence secondary to urethral atrophy is exchange of the pressure-regulating bal-loon. It is hypothesized that this may be successful due to laxity in the reservoir, which may develop over time [6]. One advantage to such an approach is avoidance of a repeat urethral dissection, which may risk urethral injury and device infection. Replacement of the reservoir with a higher-pressure reservoir is not recommended as this may increase the risk of erosion [15].

Several further adjunctive techniques have also been described in the management of recurrent SUI secondary to urethral atrophy in patients with multiple prior AUS failures. One such strategy is increasing the underlying urethral tissue bulk by placement of a small intestinal submucosal urethral wrap [26, 27] (Fig. 9.5). In two small series adequate outcomes were obtained, though

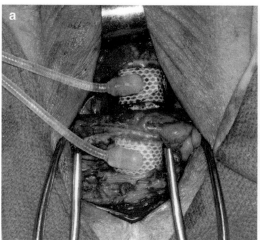 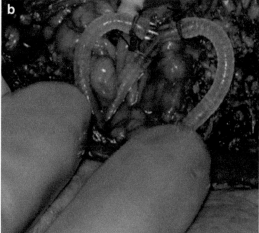

Fig. 9.4 Tandem urethral cuff placement (**a**), connection of tandem urethral cuff to in situ system (**b**)

Fig. 9.5 Intraoperative image of urethral bulking with submucosal intestinal wrap prior to AUS cuff placement

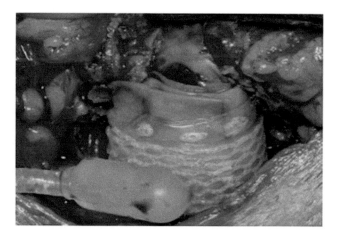

patients remained at higher risk for erosion and device failure [26, 27]. Additionally, in a small series, placement of a urethral sling proximally for additional compression in cases of urethral atrophy from an AUS has been reported [13].

Mechanical Failure

As with any prosthetic device, recurrent incontinence secondary to device malfunction may occur over time. In one series, revision for malfunction cases accounted for 25 % of revision surgeries [15]. Device malfunction can be identified on physical exam with improper device cycling and lack of coaptation of the urethral mucosa during cystoscopy. In addition, imaging with either an abdominal X-ray (if contrast was used to fill the system) or ultrasound (if normal saline was used) will confirm the diagnosis [4, 5].

Surgical management in these cases is dependent on the timing of the initial AUS placement. While no universal consensus exists, most reports suggest that when undergoing surgery for device malfunction, removal and replacement of an isolated component may be considered within 3 years of the initial implantation [6, 16]. If the device has been in situ longer than 3 years, or there is concern about other component function, removal and replacement of all components can be considered. Evaluation of additional components can be performed with intraoperative fluoroscopy and contrast instillation, use of a pressure transducer or by aspirating and measuring the fluid in the balloon [28]. Previous testing of methods for evaluating hydraulic leakage demonstrated inaccuracies with volume, pressure or electric conductance measurements for AUS devices and recommended visual evaluation of the components. Notably, this series did not evaluate the use of contrast in the device and intraoperative fluoroscopy, which is our preferred method.

A few technical considerations during AUS revision for malfunction are worth noting. First, we typically begin these cases with the perineal dissection and evaluation of the indwelling urethral cuff. This is performed first as the urethral cuff is the most commonly reported site of device malfunction [7, 16]. Dissection is carried directly on to the urethral cuff in order to exposure the cuff in its entirety and the perineal portion of the tubing. The urethral cuff is removed and tested with saline injection. The periurethral dissection is preserved with a Penrose drain which is placed around the urethral. If a leak is found from the urethral cuff, this component is replaced and reconnected to the in situ pump and reservoir via the Quick-Connect fastener (Fig. 9.6a). If no leak is detected the cuff is removed and dissection proceeds with evaluation of the abdominal reservoir and pump (Fig. 9.6b). When the abdominal components are evaluated, we tend to replace the entire device as the dissection has already been completed. One important technical consideration is ensuring the replacement of fluid in the system when replacing a single component. In these cases, we determine the volume that needs to be added based on the preoperative X-ray (presence/absence of residual contrast) and confirm with intraoperative imaging.

With regard to outcomes for revision for either mechanical failure or urethral atrophy, several series have found results comparable to primary AUS implantation [15, 29]. In the series by Raj et al. 5-year device durability was demonstrated in 80 % of primary and 88 % of secondary AUS implantations [15]. Likewise, excellent function outcomes were demonstrated, with 90 % of primary and 82 % of secondary AUS placements using zero to one pad [15].

Urethral Erosion/Device Infection

One of the most worrisome complications of AUS placement is device infection/erosion, which has been reported in 0.46–9.5 % of primary implantations [7, 30, 31]. Typically, these entities are identified through a combination of history and physical exam demonstrating signs or symptoms concerning for underlying abscess/infection, and/or evidence of urethral erosion on cystoscopy.

Device infection and erosion may be encountered from unrecognized intraoperative injury or contamination, postoperative wound infection,

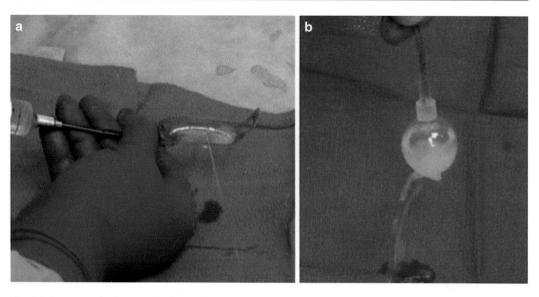

Fig. 9.6 Intraoperative image of device malfunction secondary to urethral cuff leak (**a**), abdominal reservoir leak (**b**)

compromised urethral tissues, hematogenous spread of bacteria during non-genitourinary procedures or other patient related factors. In one report, the most common organisms isolated at time of device explantation for infection were *Staphylococcus aureus, Staphylococcus epidermidis,* and gram-negative bacilli [32]. In these settings, patients should undergo reoperation with explantation of all device components, as they are considered infected/contaminated. In cases of urethral erosion, management of the site of urethral erosion has typically been via indwelling urethral Foley catheter, though recently ventral urethroplasty at the time of explantation, in an attempt to decrease stricture formation, has been reported [10, 33–35]. Following acute management, the catheter is left in place for several weeks to allow for adequate healing. In these cases, we prefer 6 weeks of postoperative catheterization with peri-catheter retrograde urethral imaging performed prior to catheter removal, to rule out persistent urethral extravasation. Notably, immediate AUS replacement following removal of an infection, non-eroded, AUS has been reported, but is not considered standard practice [36].

Following repeat evaluation 4–6 months after device explantation for infection or erosion, salvage AUS implantation may be considered. This evaluation should include history, physical exami-

nation, urinalysis, post-void residual and cystoscopy to rule out urethral stricture. If adequate urethral healing has occurred and the patient wishes to proceed, reimplantation can be considered. Notably, these are difficult reoperative cases secondary to scarring and loss of tissue planes from the previous inflammation and infection. With repeat perineal dissection we attempt to avoid excessive mobilization of the urethra in an effort to preserve already tenuous blood supply. Depending on the tissue quality, an adequate location for cuff placement is determined. In many of these cases, a transcorporal approach is needed secondary to compromised urethral tissue or obliterated dissection planes [10, 20, 22] (Fig. 9.7). Notably, preservation of erectile function with use of the transcorporal approach has been reported [37]. Lastly, as with all AUS placements, evaluation of urethral integrity following periurethral dissection (either via cystoscopy or pericatheter fluid injection) is needed.

In contrast to cases of AUS revision for atrophy or mechanical failure, reimplantation following device erosion or infection has been associated with an increased risk of repeat explantation [10, 29, 38, 39]. This finding is intuitive given the technical challenges and typically poor tissue quality encountered in these cases. Notably, however, even in this setting, reasonable long-term

Fig. 9.7 Intraoperative image of transcorporal AUS cuff placement

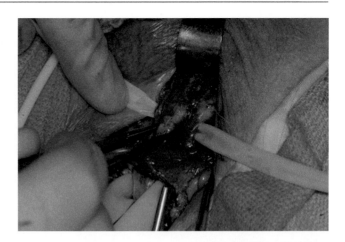

device survival has been reported [10, 29, 38, 39]. In fact, in the largest series on salvage AUS reimplantation, similar 5-year device survival was found between primary and reimplantation cases after an infection or erosion event (76 % versus 68 %). One strategy to avoid further urethral atrophy and potential repeat erosion in the setting of compromised urethral tissue is nightly device deactivation [40].

Given that many patients experience severe recurrent urinary incontinence after device explantation, and the dramatic impact on quality of life this can have, salvage AUS reimplantation can be considered. However, patient counseling regarding the increased risk of recurrent infection/ erosion is needed.

Other Considerations

A potential etiology for persistent incontinence following AUS placement is improper location of cuff placement or inaccurate urethral sizing. Both of these can be identified during evaluation with physical exam and office cystoscopy. Optimal cuff location is at the proximal aspect of the bulbar urethra. In order to adequately expose this area, we prefer a perineal approach as opposed to a penoscrotal approach, which we feel may lead to a more distal placement. Appropriate cuff placement (further proximal) is demonstrated in a patient referred for management of persistent incontinence after transscrotal AUS placement (Fig. 9.8).

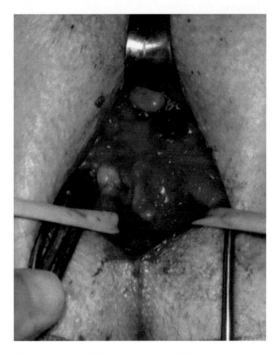

Fig. 9.8 Malpositioned urethral cuff in distal urethral location encountered during AUS revision. Seen is a penrose drain placed around the new cuff location in the proximal bulbar urethra

One additional unique scenario for recurrent incontinence following AUS placement is patients that have suffered a decrease in cognition or manual dexterity since their initial AUS placement. These patients may have recurrent incontinence secondary to improper device utilization and overflow incontinence. In certain instances, this may be managed with device deactivation and symptomatic management of the resultant incontinence. However, in some cases, device deactivation or removal with male urethral sling placement could be considered.

Anti-incontinence Surgery Following a Failed Urethral Sling

Due to a desire to avoid a mechanical device and the attendant risks of device malfunction or erosion, as well as the need for device manipulation, many men prefer urethral sling placement, even when not considered ideal candidates [41]. However, for optimal outcomes for male urethral sling placement, patient selection is crucial. In that regard, several factors have been associated with increased rates of persistent stress urinary incontinence including pad weight greater than 450 g per day, previous pelvic radiation therapy and a low detrusor leak point pressure [8].

For patients with persistent or recurrent stress incontinence after male urethral sling placement, revision surgery either via repeat urethral sling or more commonly artificial urinary sphincter placement has been reported. In this setting, placement of an AUS is typically utilized as the presence of fibrosis hinders urethral compression and/or mobility, which are crucial for sling efficacy [8, 12, 14].

Several reports have demonstrated, albeit in small series, excellent outcomes for AUS placement after a previous urethral sling [42–44]. For instance, in a series of 28 patients undergoing AUS after a failed urethral sling, similar high success rates with limited complications were seen when compared to a control group without prior urethral sling surgery [42]. In our experience, in the majority of cases of AUS placement in patients with a prior urethral sling, the sling can be left in situ without need for excision. If the sling is encountered we prefer to incise the sling rather than perform urethrolysis, as this risks urethral injury, as well potentially compromising urethral blood supply.

Despite previous sling failure, for a variety of reasons, some patients opt for a repeat urethral sling placement rather than AUS implantation. In a series of 35 cases of repeat transobturator urethral sling placement, 76 % of patients were dry or using a security pad at 6-month follow up [45]. In their experience, removal of the previous sling was unnecessary as the previous sling was not in the appropriate position, which may indicate prior sling slippage [45].

Conclusions

Regardless of the type of primary anti-incontinence surgery, revision surgery for post-prostatectomy incontinence is a relatively common entity. For patients with a prior AUS, this may be in the form of revision for atrophy, malfunction or erosion. In the case of atrophy and malfunction, completed device exchange is typically performed if initial implantation was 3 years or prior, with exchange of a single component in other cases. When erosion is encountered, explantation of all components, with potential delayed reimplantation considered, though this can be technically challenging. In patients with persistent or recurrent SUI after male urethral sling placement, limited data is available. From the series available, AUS placement may provide excellent outcomes, though repeat urethral sling placement can be considered if the previous sling has slipped from initial placement as seen during repositioning on office cystoscopy.

References

1. Van Der Aa F, Drake MJ, Kasyan GR, Petrolekas A. The artificial urinary sphincter after a quarter of a century: a critical systematic review of its use in male non-neurogenic incontinence. Eur Urol. 2013;63:681–9.
2. Trost L, Elliott DS. Male stress urinary incontinence: a review of surgical treatment options and outcomes. Adv Urol. 2012;2012:287489.
3. Gormley EA, Lightner DJ, Burgio KL, et al. Diagnosis and treatment of overactive bladder (non-neurogenic) in adults: AUA/SUFU guideline. J Urol. 2012;188: 2455–63.
4. Petrou SP, Williams HJJR, Young PR. Radiographic imaging of the artificial urinary sphincter pressure regulating balloon. J Urol. 2001;165:1773–5.

5. Brucker BM, Demirtas A, Fong E, Kelly C, Nitti VW. Artificial urinary sphincter revision: the role of ultrasound. Urology. 2013;82:1424–8.
6. Wang R, McGuire EJ, He C, Faerber GJ, Latini JM. Long-term outcomes after primary failures of artificial urinary sphincter implantation. Urology. 2012; 79:922–8.
7. Lai HH, Hsu EI, Teh BS, Butler EB, Boone TB. 13 years of experience with artificial urinary sphincter implantation at Baylor College of Medicine. J Urol. 2007;177:1021–5.
8. Jura YH, Comiter CV. Urodynamics for postprostatectomy incontinence: when are they helpful and how do we use them? Urol Clin North Am. 2014;41: 419–27.
9. Bauer RM, Gozzi C, Roosen A, et al. Impact of the "repositioning test" on postoperative outcome of retroluminar transobturator male sling implantation. Urol Int. 2013;90:334–8.
10. Linder BJ, de Cogain M, Elliott DS. Long-term device outcomes of artificial urinary sphincter reimplantation following prior explantation for erosion or infection. J Urol. 2014;191:734–8.
11. Kim SP, Sarmast Z, Daignault S, Faerber GJ, McGuire EJ, Latini JM. Long-term durability and functional outcomes among patients with artificial urinary sphincters: a 10-year retrospective review from the University of Michigan. J Urol. 2008;179:1912–6.
12. Tuygun C, Imamoglu A, Gucuk A, Goktug G, Demirel F. Comparison of outcomes for adjustable bulbourethral male sling and artificial urinary sphincter after previous artificial urinary sphincter erosion. Urology. 2009;73:1363–7.
13. Christine B, Knoll LD. Treatment of recurrent urinary incontinence after artificial urinary sphincter placement using the AdVance male sling. Urology. 2010;76:1321–4.
14. Tuygun C, Imamoglu A, Keyik B, Alisir I, Yorubulut M. Significance of fibrosis around and/or at external urinary sphincter on pelvic magnetic resonance imaging in patients with postprostatectomy incontinence. Urology. 2006;68:1308–12.
15. Raj GV, Peterson AC, Toh KL, Webster GD. Outcomes following revisions and secondary implantation of the artificial urinary sphincter. J Urol. 2005;173:1242–5.
16. Webster GD, Sherman ND. Management of male incontinence following artificial urinary sphincter failure. Curr Opin Urol. 2005;15:386–90.
17. Saffarian A, Walsh K, Walsh IK, Stone AR. Urethral atrophy after artificial urinary sphincter placement: is cuff downsizing effective? J Urol. 2003;169:567–9.
18. Hudak SJ, Morey AF. Impact of 3.5 cm artificial urinary sphincter cuff on primary and revision surgery for male stress urinary incontinence. J Urol. 2011;186: 1962–6.
19. Simhan J, Morey AF, Singla N, et al. 3.5 cm artificial urinary sphincter cuff erosion occurs predominantly in radiated patients. J Urol. 2014. doi:10.1016/j. juro.2014.07.115.
20. Guralnick ML, Miller E, Toh KL, Webster GD. Transcorporal artificial urinary sphincter cuff placement in cases requiring revision for erosion and urethral atrophy. J Urol. 2002;167:2075–8.
21. Brito CG, Mulcahy JJ, Mitchell ME, Adams MC. Use of a double cuff AMS800 urinary sphincter for severe stress incontinence. J Urol. 1993;149:283–5.
22. Magera JS, Elliott DS. Tandem transcorporal artificial urinary sphincter cuff salvage technique: surgical description and results. J Urol. 2007;177:1015–9.
23. DiMarco DS, Elliott DS. Tandem cuff artificial urinary sphincter as a salvage procedure following failed primary sphincter placement for the treatment of post-prostatectomy incontinence. J Urol. 2003; 170:1252–4.
24. O'Connor RC, Lyon MB, Guralnick ML, Bales GT. Long-term follow-up of single versus double cuff artificial urinary sphincter insertion for the treatment of severe postprostatectomy stress urinary incontinence. Urology. 2008;71:90–3.
25. Kowalczyk JJ, Spicer DL, Mulcahy JJ. Erosion rate of the double cuff AMS800 artificial urinary sphincter: long-term followup. J Urol. 1996;156:1300–1.
26. Trost L, Elliott D. Small intestinal submucosa urethral wrap at the time of artificial urinary sphincter placement as a salvage treatment option for patients with persistent/recurrent incontinence following multiple prior sphincter failures and erosions. Urology. 2012;79:933–8.
27. Rahman NU, Minor TX, Deng D, Lue TF. Combined external urethral bulking and artificial urinary sphincter for urethral atrophy and stress urinary incontinence. BJU Int. 2005;95:824–6.
28. Chung E, Cartmill R. Diagnostic challenges in the evaluation of persistent or recurrent urinary incontinence after artificial urinary sphincter (AUS) implantation in patients after prostatectomy. BJU Int. 2013;112:32–5.
29. Lai HH, Boone TB. Complex artificial urinary sphincter revision and reimplantation cases--how do they fare compared to virgin cases? J Urol. 2012;187:951–5.
30. Elliott DS, Barret DM. Mayo clinic long-term analysis of the functional durability of the AMS 800 artificial urinary sphincter: a review of 323 cases. J Urol. 1998;159:1206–8.
31. Montague DK, Angermeier KW. Artificial urinary sphincter troubleshooting. Urology. 2001;58:779–82.
32. Magera JS, Elliott DS. Artificial urinary sphincter infection: causative organisms in a contemporary series. J Urol. 2008;180:2475–8.
33. Kowalczyk JJ, Nelson R, Mulcahy JJ. Successful reinsertion of the artificial urinary sphincter after removal for erosion or infection. Urology. 1996;48:906–8.
34. Flynn BJ, Webster GD. Evaluation and surgical. Rev Urol. 2004;6:180–6.
35. Rozanski AT, Tausch TJ, Ramirez D, Simhan J, Scott JF, Morey AF. Immediate urethral repair during explantation prevents stricture formation after artificial urinary sphincter cuff erosion. J Urol. 2014;192(2):442–6.

36. Bryan DE, Mulcahy JJ, Simmons GR. Salvage procedure for infected noneroded artificial urinary sphincters. J Urol. 2002;168:2464–6.
37. Wiedemann L, Cornu J-N, Haab E, et al. Transcorporal artificial urinary sphincter implantation as a salvage surgical procedure for challenging cases of male stress urinary incontinence: surgical technique and functional outcomes in a contemporary series. BJU Int. 2013;112:1163–8.
38. Frank I, Elliott DS, Barrett DM. Success of de novo reimplantation of the artificial genitourinary sphincter. J Urol. 2000;163:1702–3.
39. Raj GV, Peterson AC, Webster GD. Outcomes following erosions of the artificial urinary sphincter. J Urol. 2006;175:2186–90. discussion 2190.
40. Elliott DS, Barrett DM, Gohma M, Boone TB. Does nocturnal deactivation of the artificial urinary sphincter lessen the risk of urethral atrophy? Urology. 2001;57:1051–4.
41. Kumar A, Litt ER, Ballert KN, Nitti VW. Artificial urinary sphincter versus male sling for post-prostatectomy incontinence—what do patients choose? J Urol. 2009;181:1231–5.
42. Lentz AC, Peterson AC, Webster GD. Outcomes following artificial sphincter implantation after prior unsuccessful male sling. J Urol. 2012;187:2149–53.
43. Fisher MB, Aggarwal N, Vuruskan H, Singla AK. Efficacy of artificial urinary sphincter implantation after failed bone-anchored male sling for postprostatectomy incontinence. Urology. 2007;70:942–4.
44. Abdou A, Cornu J-N, Sèbe P, et al. Salvage therapy with artificial urinary sphincter after Advance™ male sling failure for post-prostatectomy incontinence: a first clinical experience. Prog Urol. 2012;22:650–6.
45. Soljanik I, Becker AJ, Stief CG, Gozzi C, Bauer RM. Repeat retrourethral transobturator sling in the management of recurrent postprostatectomy stress urinary incontinence after failed first male sling. Eur Urol. 2010;58:767–72.

Part III

Adverse Events After Radiotherapy

Post-RT Urinary Incontinence and Stricture

10

Gillian Stearns and Laura Leddy

Introduction

Prostate cancer is the most common solid organ malignancy in men with an estimated 220,800 new diagnoses in the USA in 2015 (SEER database seer.cancer.gov). Radiation therapy (RT) as a treatment for prostate cancer began in 1904 when Imbert and Imbert used radiation to treat a patient with advanced disease. It has been used in the USA since 1915 [1]. Based on 2007 SEER database results, 20 % of men who are newly diagnosed with prostate cancer select external beam radiotherapy (EBRT), 10 % select brachytherapy (BT) and 4 % receive a combination of BT and EBRT (Elliot SP, Jarosek SA, Virnig BA, written communication, October 2011). The AUA guidelines offer radiotherapy as a treatment option for low, moderate and high risk prostate cancer, although recurrence rates increase when radiation is used as monotherapy for high risk disease [2]. While cure rates are excellent for low and moderate risk prostate cancer, there are several known urinary complications that can result

from the use of radiotherapy in treatment of prostate cancer. This chapter discusses post-RT urinary incontinence and post-RT urethral stricture disease.

Section I: Post-RT Urinary Incontinence

Pathophysiology of Post-RT Urinary Incontinence

Urinary incontinence after the treatment of localized prostate cancer is primarily discussed in the setting of post-prostatectomy stress urinary incontinence (SUI). Urinary incontinence associated with radiotherapy for localized prostate cancer is discussed much less frequently. Radiotherapy for prostate cancer can result in lower urinary tract symptoms (LUTS) that manifest as both irritative symptoms and storage symptoms. In their severe form the storage symptoms can result in overactive bladder (OAB) and urgency urinary incontinence [3]. OAB is a combination of storage symptoms including urgency, frequency and nocturia with or without urgency urinary incontinence [4]. OAB is caused by involuntary contractions of the detrusor muscle during the filing phase of the bladder, a time when the detrusor should be relaxed and compliant [5].

Voiding dysfunction following radiotherapy for prostate cancer is divided into early and late phases. The pathophysiology of early bladder

G. Stearns, M.D.
Department of Urology, University of Vermont, Burlington, VT, USA

L. Leddy, M.D. (✉)
Department of Surgery, Urology Service, Memorial Sloan Kettering Cancer Center, 353 E 68 St., New York, NY 10065, USA
e-mail: leddyl@mskcc.org

© Springer International Publishing Switzerland 2016
J.S. Sandhu (ed.), *Urinary Dysfunction in Prostate Cancer*, DOI 10.1007/978-3-319-23817-3_10

dysfunction following radiation is not clearly understood. Two possible mechanisms for the early phase bladder dysfunction have been suggested. The first suggests smooth muscle edema may be the cause [6]. The second theory for early post-RT voiding dysfunction relates to inflammation and injury to the urothelium. On microscopic examination, hyperemia and scattered degeneration is noted on urothelial biopsy specimens in the days to weeks following radiation [7]. Urodynamic studies performed in an animal model 14 days following irradiation show a decreased compliance, which resolved over the following 2–4 weeks. The severity of this decreased compliance is proportional to the radiotherapy dose [8]. Changes in innervation do not appear to be associated with this early phase bladder dysfunction [7].

The late bladder dysfunction appears to be the result of vascular changes and fibrosis, which lead to a decrease in bladder capacity [7, 9]. After the initiation of radiotherapy, edema results, followed by fibrosis, and disorganization of the bladder wall during the 6–12 months that follow radiotherapy. At the bladder neck, perivascular fibrosis leads to vascular occlusion and ischemia, ultimately resulting in fibrosis at the bladder neck. This fibrosis may result in decreased compliance and functional as well as anatomic changes in bladder capacity [7]. Choo et al. performed urodyamic studies on 17 patients both prior to EBRT and 18 months following EBRT. They found a significant reduction in bladder capacity of an average of 100 mL at 18 months following EBRT as well as a significant reduction in the volume at first sensation and the volume at which subjects desired to void [9]. During the late phase bladder sensation may also be altered due to changes in the innervation of the trigone [3].

The OAB and urgency urinary incontinence that occurs after radiotherapy for prostate cancer may be the result of these changes to the bladder mucosa, detrusor innervation and bladder neck. In a minority of patients, post-RT urinary incontinence is the result of overflow incontinence, due to prostatic obstruction, urethral stricture or detrusor under activity. Urethral stricture will be discussed later in this chapter.

Prevalence of Post-RT Urinary Incontinence

An understanding of the pretreatment prevalence of urinary incontinence is important in order to understand the posttreatment burden of disease. Markland et al. using the NHANES database found the overall risk of urinary incontinence was 14 % in American men aged >20 years with time and race-dependent variation [10]. Litwin et al. found a 6 % rate of severe urinary incontinence, defined as no urinary control or frequent leakage in elderly men without prostate cancer [11]. Resnick et al. found between 5 and 9 % of prostate cancer patients report pretreatment severe urinary incontinence with 7 % reporting "frequent dribbling or no urinary control" and 17 % reporting urinary leakage at least once per day or more [12]. The risk of pretreatment urinary incontinence is directly related to patient comorbidities, with 6 % of patients with TIBI-CaP scores from 0 to 2 suffering from urinary incontinence while 21 % of patients with a TIBI-CaP score >9 suffering from pretreatment urinary incontinence ($P<0.001$) [12]. The EPIC study evaluated the baseline prevalence of OAB within five western countries of urgency (19 %), frequency (11 %), urgency incontinence (2.5 %) [13]. Based on these varied studies the prevalence of pretreatment urinary incontinence varies dramatically by age and comorbidities from as low as 2.5 % to as high as 21 % in some populations. It should be noted, however, that most patients who are candidates for contemporary RT are well screened for LUTS and urinary incontinence and those that are at a high risk for urinary adverse events are often not offered RT.

The prevalence of post-RT urinary incontinence varies based on the definition of urinary incontinence, treatment modality and time from therapy. The Prostate Cancer Outcomes Study estimated that the prevalence of urinary incontinence is 4 % and 9.4 % in all patients 5 years and 15 years after radiotherapy for prostate cancer [14]. While Sanda et al. found a patient-reported incidence of post-RT urinary incontinence in 4–6 % of men with persistent incontinence at 1–2 years [15]. In a cross sectional study of 102 patients, with a median follow up of 5.2 years post-brachytherapy, 45 % of men reported incontinence. Only 16 % of those required daily pad usage, with 11 % reporting a few drops, and another 11 % reporting daily leakage not requiring pad usage [16]. Blaivas et al. found an elevated incidence of OAB symptoms (79 %), detrusor overactivity on urodynamics (85 %), and urinary incontinence (71 %) in men with symptomatic LUTS 6 months after brachytherapy for localized prostate cancer [17]. This predominance of DO and urgency urinary incontinence in post-RT patients is underscored by a SEER study of 5621 older men after BT for prostate cancer, 7.5 % reported urinary incontinence greater than 2 years after therapy, while 0.2 % received an invasive procedure for the incontinence [18]. Choo et al., however, did not find any difference in bladder compliance, bladder stability or bladder outlet flow on urodynamic evaluation before and 18 months after EBRT in their quantitative study of 17 patients despite a measurable and significant change in bladder capacity [9].

Combination BT and EBRT is associated with a higher rate of urinary incontinence. In a review of the SEER database, 1915, 1893, and 555 patients underwent external beam therapy, brachytherapy and combined therapy, respectively. Combined modality therapy resulted in incontinence rates of 56.8 % versus 49.1 % for BT alone and 29.2 % for EBRT alone [19].

There is some evidence that post-RT urinary incontinence may improve with time. Sanda et al. performed a prospective, multicenter analysis of men with localized prostate cancer who underwent surgery, brachytherapy or external beam radiotherapy. 1201 patients were followed for 24 months. In patients who received EBRT alone, urinary symptoms, including incontinence had resolved by 12 months, additionally patients reported LUTS were improved over baseline at 24 months. In the BT cohort; however at 24 months, patients had not returned to baseline [15].

Evaluation of Post-RT Urinary Incontinence

The evaluation of post-RT urinary incontinence begins with a focused history, noting in particular: preoperative voiding dysfunction and urinary incontinence, the status of the current cancer treatment and plans for future therapy and surveillance, medical comorbidities and prior pelvic surgery. Validated questionnaires are a helpful adjunct to the medical history. The International Prostate Symptom Score (IPSS) can be used to objectively score and compare LUTS during therapy for symptoms. The focused physical examination confirms stress urinary incontinence and evaluates for anatomic or neurologic abnormalities [20]. Diagnostic and laboratory evaluation should include urine analysis and urine culture with proper evaluation of hematuria (cystoscopy and CT or MR urogram) and treatment of urinary tract infection should they exist. Uroflowmetry and a post-void residual allow for the differentiation of overflow incontinence due to bladder outlet obstruction or urethral stricture, from stress or urgency urinary incontinence. A 72-h voiding diary and 24 h pad weight test allows for objective information on the volume and timing of leakage, functional bladder capacity and consumption of bladder irritants. The voiding diary is a useful tool for linking behavior to leakage. Urodynamic studies confirm the diagnosis of urge and/or stress urinary incontinence, detrusor overactivity, and bladder capacity. The study also quantifies detrusor contraction strength which is often diminished with increasing age and pelvic radiation [21]. The AUA/SUFU guidelines recommend evaluation of urgency urinary incontinence to evaluate if there is a component of bladder outlet obstruction that may be exacerbating detrusor overactivity [22]. Cystoscopic evaluation rules out urethral stricture and confirms sphincter contractility as well as intravesical disease.

Medical Management of Urgency Urinary Incontinence

Initial management of OAB due to DO and resulting in urgency urinary incontinence in the post-RT patient should involve counseling regarding behavioral modification based on information gained from the patient's voiding diary. Once a reduction in bladder irritants and fluid consumption in the hours prior to sleep has occurred medical therapy is initiated as needed.

Multiple studies have demonstrated the effectiveness of alpha-blockers in reducing urinary toxicity after radiotherapy treatment. Their proposed mechanism of efficacy is a reduction in trigonal hyperactivity and a decrease in overall bladder irritability [23]. Zelefsky et al. evaluated 743 patients between 1988 and 1995 who underwent EBRT. Grade 2 urinary toxicity was witnessed in 37 % of patients (275). Terazosin was given to 119 of the 275 patients with bothersome symptoms. 79 reported a "significant" response as compared to 11 reporting the same response after receiving NSAID treatment. Younger patients (less than 65) tended to report a greater improvement. Clinical stage and preoperative voiding dysfunction was not found to be significantly different between the responders and non-responders [24].

Elshaikh et al. evaluated the use of tamsulosin in patients undergoing BT for localized prostate cancer. 126 patients underwent a randomized, double-blinded study evaluating the use of tamsulosin 0.8 mg versus placebo. Patients were instructed to begin tamsulosin 4 days prior to seed implant. AUA symptom score was given weekly for the first 8 weeks following implant to evaluate change in symptoms. 82 patients completed the trial. By week five the tamsulosin group had a significant reduction in AUA score versus placebo. This difference persisted throughout the remaining 3 weeks. Peak urinary morbidity was reported between week 2 and 3, patients should be counseled to expect this following BT [23].

The DO and urgency urinary incontinence associated with radiotherapy for prostate cancer is associated with irritative lower urinary symptoms. Oral anticholinergic therapy has been evaluated for possible management of these urinary symptoms. Bittner et al. evaluated 69 patients who underwent brachytherapy from 1999 to 2005 and provided trospium for patients presenting with irritative symptoms. Patients received medication at a median of 23.4 months after implantation. Pre-implantation mean IPSS was 6.5. At the time of medication initiation, mean IPSS was 9.5. IPSS resolved to baseline in 55/69 patients (77 %) with anticholinergic therapy. Median follow-up was 38 months. 22/69 discontinued trospium secondary

to side effects or resolution of symptoms. Primary side effects included retention, constipation, and dry mouth [25]. In an appropriately selected patient, anticholinergics may help with irritative voiding symptoms. A post-void residual and uroflowmetry should be performed prior to initiation of anticholinergic therapy due to the risk of urinary retention with these medications.

Beta-3 agonists are becoming increasingly common in the treatment of OAB and urgency urinary incontinence [26, 27]. However, their use has not been studied for post-RT LUTS. A trial of a beta-3 agonist is warranted in the patient with OAB and urgency urinary incontinence after RT in lieu of or addition to anticholinergic therapy.

Third-Line Therapies for Post-RT Urinary Incontinence

The OAB associated with RT for prostate cancer generally improves with time. For the minority of patients with persistent, severe post-RT LUTS, refractory to pharmacologic therapy, third-line therapies for OAB and urgency urinary incontinence such as botulinum toxin A or sacral nerve stimulation can be considered. As a final option, urinary diversion is offered to well-counseled patients who have failed all other options.

Conclusions

The reported prevalence of post-RT urinary incontinence is as high as 50–80 %, depending on the time from treatment and the treatment modality, with the majority being caused by detrusor overactivity. Pretreatment and posttreatment with alpha-blockade can improve post-RT urinary symptoms. Persistent post-RT urinary incontinence is evaluated and managed in a similar fashion to patients with idiopathic urgency urinary incontinence. Particular attention is paid to the known changes in detrusor and bladder neck function that occur after radiotherapy, to the possibility of persistent or recurrent malignancy and to the possibility of anatomic obstruction secondary to a post-RT urethral stricture.

Section II: Post- RT Urethral Stricture

Pathophysiology of Urethral Stricture Formation

The male urethra passes through the prostate making portions of the urethra susceptible to radiation-induced injury during RT for prostate cancer. Radiation damages the deoxyribonucleic acid in actively dividing cells causing oxidative stress and cell death, this leads to the therapeutic effect of radiation therapy but can also lead to the adverse effect of progressive endarteritis in sub-mucosal and muscular tissues [28, 29]. In this setting wound healing becomes compromised leading to atrophy, contraction and permanent fibrosis [30]. The end product of this is post-RT urethral stricture disease.

Incidence of Urethral Stricture Formation by Modality

The incidence of post-RT urethral stricture disease varies by radiation modality and time from radiation administration leading to wide variability in the reported incidence within the literature. Additionally, the reported incidence may under-estimate rates of urethral stricture disease after radiotherapy as only those cases that cause enough symptoms to warrant urologic evaluation will be diagnosed [31, 32].

The rates of urethral stricture after BT range from 0 to 10.2 % with 23–63 months of follow up [33–37]. Similar rates of urethral stricture are reported in several series of high-dose-rate brachytherapy with stricture rates of 7–8 % at 5 year follow up [38, 39]. One series found a 30 % incidence of urethral stricture in patients who received 19Gy in two treatments vs. 3.4 % and 2.3 % for 18Gy/3 and 20Gy/4 respectively. This finding prompted a change in BT administration technique. [40] The reported incidence of urethral stricture after EBRT increases depending on length of follow up with an incidence of less than 7 % with 5 years of follow up and growing to 10–18 % when follow up is increased up to 10 years [36, 41–44]. The

CaPSURE database presented urethral stricture rates by radiation modality as follows brachytherapy (1.8 %), EBRT (1.7 %), combination RT (5.2 %) with a median follow up of 2.7 years [32].

In two small series the incidence of posterior urethral stricture after adjuvant or salvage EBRT was 3 and 9 % at 5 and 2 years of follow up respectively [45, 46]. This incidence would likely increase with further follow up.

Location of Radiation Therapy Induced Urethral Stricture Formation

Greater than 90 % of post-RT urethral strictures occur in the bulbomembranous urethra [35, 39]. While the bulbomembranous urethral is distal to the apex of the prostate it is relatively exposed resulting in its risk for injury. Several studies have demonstrated the incidence of radiotherapy induced bulbomembraous urethral stricture was related to the radiotherapy dose delivered to the prostatic apex. [33, 37] In a SEER study of 5621 men who underwent BT from 1991 to 1999, Chen et al. found that while urinary morbidity following brachytherapy was common, the rate of post-RT procedures declined during the 1990s suggesting improvements in RT delivery during the decade that led to fewer cases of post-RT urinary obstruction [18].

Urethral Stricture: Presentation and Diagnosis

The presentation of post-RT urethral stricture disease ranges from asymptomatic to acute urinary retention and includes irritative lower urinary tract symptoms such as frequency, urgency and urge or stress urinary incontinence and obstructive lower urinary tract symptoms such as weak stream, incomplete emptying and overflow incontinence [47]. The diagnosis of post-RT urethral stricture disease is complicated by the incidence of post-RT LUTS unrelated to urethral stenosis.

Patients with persistent or worsening lower urinary tract symptoms after the completion of radiotherapy, gross hematuria and acute urinary retention should be evaluated by an urologist. Given that post-RT urethral strictures occur in as many as a one in ten patients after older forms of radiotherapy for prostate cancer, urologists should keep the diagnosis in mind when evaluating post-RT patients with LUTS or an elevated post-void residual measurement.

Evaluation

The need for the evaluation of post-RT LUTS is determined by the severity and duration of the symptoms. [31] As indicated above, the history may include a worsening of irritative and/or obstructive LUTS symptoms as well as worsening urinary incontinence.

The evaluation of post-RT LUTS includes a medical history evaluating the progress of the prostate cancer treatment, pretreatment and post-treatment LUTS and urinary incontinence as well as the patient's goals of treatment. Validated questionnaires are a helpful adjunct to the medical history. The International Prostate Symptom Score (IPSS) can be used to objectively score and compare LUTS during therapy for symptoms.

The physical examination should include a general examination, as well as examination of the abdomen, genitals, digital rectal and perineum. Abdominal examination may reveal a distended bladder in the setting of urinary retention. Digital rectal examination typically reveals a small, flattened prostate. On genital examination the meatus is not typically involved in the post-RT related urethral stricture disease, however, meatal stenosis unrelated to treatment, can cause similar symptoms. Laboratory evaluation should include a PSA, urinalysis and urine culture with appropriate evaluation and treatment of hematuria and/or urinary tract infection if present. Consider renal function testing, especially in the setting of an elevated post-void residual or urinary retention.

In office diagnostic studies include uroflowmetry to assess for a blunted flow curve, suggesting urethral obstruction, a valsalva pattern suggesting detrusor weakness, and a post-void residual measurement to assess for urinary retention due to obstruction or detrusor failure. Cystoscopy is indicated in patients with microscopic or gross hematuria and should be considered in the evaluation of post-RT patients with an elevated post void residual, peak flow less than 12 cc/s with a flattened uroflowmetry curve and LUTS that are markedly worse than pretreatment and unaffected by oral alpha-blockade. Flexible cystoscopy, using a 16Fr cystoscope, provides a definitive diagnosis of urethral stricture as well as bladder stones, bladder tumors, obstructing prostatic lobes and some measure of external sphincter coaptation and function. Urodynamic evaluation is less helpful in the setting of a urethral stricture, however, can be helpful in the evaluation of post-RT LUTS as described above.

Urethral Imaging Techniques

Urethral imaging can be performed via retrograde urethrogram (RUG) and voiding cystourethrogram (VCUG) or with urethral ultrasound. The combination of the RUG and VCUG allows for evaluation of the length, location and caliber of the urethral stricture, all factors important for preoperative planning (Fig. 10.1).

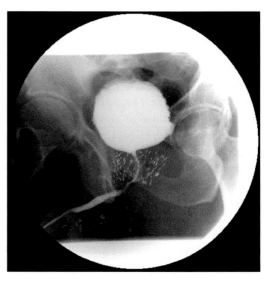

Fig. 10.1 Diagnostic RUG/VCUG demonstrates bulbo-membranous urethral stricture. Brachytherapy seeds are present within the prostate

Urethral ultrasound is typically performed under anesthesia prior to urethral repair by placing the ultrasound probe on the perineum while instilling normal saline into the meatus via a 60 mL catheter tip syringe and applying gentle suprapubic pressure. Urethral ultrasound avoids radiation and allows for evaluation of the length, location and caliber of the urethral stricture as well as the degree of fibrosis within the corpus spongiosum.

Endoscopic Management of Radiated Urethral Stricture

Initial management of radiated strictures in the bulbomembranous and bulbar urethra is often similar to non-radiated urethral strictures in the same anatomic location. In general, a trial of endoscopic management with dilation, direct vision internal urethrotomy (DVIU) or laser urethrotomy is performed. Limited information is published on the outcomes of endoscopic management of post-RT urethral stricture disease. Merrick et al. described 29 patients treated with either dilation or DVIU after the diagnosis of a brachytherapy induced urethral stricture, 31 % (9/29) required repeat endoscopic procedures with 10 % (3/29) eventually requiring a suprapubic tube and the other 21 % (6/29) maintaining urethral patency with intermittent self catheterization (IC). Unfortunately, no follow up information is available for the remaining patients in the series [35].

Repeat endoscopic management of radiated urethral strictures can be performed. Patients should be counseled that repeat endoscopic treatments are rarely a definitive treatment. Patients require continued surveillance in order to prevent bladder and eventually renal dysfunction from recurrent urethral stenosis.

Little is published on the recommended follow up for patients after either initial or repeat endoscopic management of post-RT urethral stricture disease. In practice, the patient generally removes the catheter between 24 and 72 h after the endoscopic procedure. A clinic visit is recommended at 3 and 12 months postoperatively with evaluation of subjective voiding symptoms, uroflowmetry, post-void residual urine measurement and cystoscopy.

Thereafter, yearly visits to evaluate subjective voiding symptoms, uroflowmetry, post-void residual urine measurement and consideration for cystoscopy if any parameters are abnormal.

Endoscopic management of post-RT urethral strictures combined with a urethral stent has been described, however, currently no urethral stent available for clinical use [48].

Operative Repair of Post-RT Urethral Strictures

The majority of post-RT urethral strictures occur in the bulbomembranous urethra. In this location, a urethroplasty is performed through a perineal incision. A midline perineal incision allows for excellent access to the bulbomembranous urethra. In cases where the stenosis extends into the prostatic urethra a lambda incision may be preferable as it improves visualization of the posterior urethra and facilitates the placement of a gracilis muscle flap.

An anastomotic technique was performed in the majority of urethroplasties performed for post-RT urethral stricture disease and described in the literature [49, 50]. In these cases, a circumferential dissection was performed at the level of the bulbomembranous urethra and the urethra was divided at the distal extent of the urethral stenosis. The dissection is carried proximally until the entire length of the stenosed urethra is resected and sent for pathologic evaluation. In some cases the stenosis extends into the apex of the prostate, necessitating a partial prostatectomy, in order to bring healthy urethral mucosa together. During this dissection brachytherapy seeds are often encountered and should be removed to facilitate the anastomosis. Significant mucosal calcification may be encountered once the urethral lumen is entered (Fig. 10.2). The scarred and calcified tissue should be fully resected and the fresh distal and proximal edges spatulated prior to urethral reconstruction. Urethral mobilization, corporal body splitting, corporal rerouting, and partial pubectomy are surgical maneuvers that may be required to create a tension-free anastomosis. In cases where a large perineal defect exists or for severe radiation

Fig. 10.2 Intraoperative photo of patient in lithotomy with perineal incision. The bulbar urethra is divided at the level of the calcified post- RT urethral stricture. The distal urethral is mobilized to the level of the penoscrotal junction to allow for a tension-free anastomosis

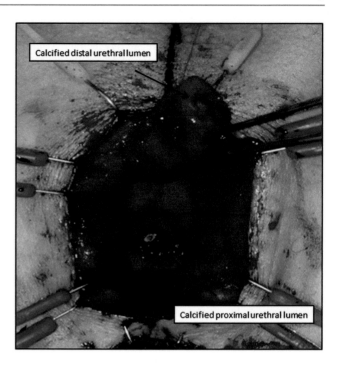

damage a gracilis muscle flap can be brought into the perineum to improve tissue healing.

The reported success of operative urethroplasty for post-RT urethral strictures ranges from 69.7 to 90 % with the majority being completed using an anastomotic technique and a mean stricture length of 2.3 cm and 2.6 cm respectively and follow up of greater than 40 months [49, 50]. A ventral onlay technique combined with a gracilis muscle flap was used in 20 patients including 9 who received radiotherapy for prostate cancer with a 77.8 % success rate for the post-RT patients and a mean stricture length of 8.2 cm and median follow up of 26.5 months [51].

Post-operative Considerations

Validated questionnaires to evaluate patient reported outcome measures (PROMS) are in development though are not included in published post-RT urethroplasty series. Two outcomes frequently evaluated in the post-operative setting after urethroplasty are continence and erectile function.

The majority of post-RT urethral strictures involve the external urinary sphincter. Anastomotic urethroplasty typically involves removal of this section of the uretha, while ventral onlay may require incising the sphincter. In both situations the patient will be relying on an intact internal urinary sphincter as the primary post-operative continence mechanism. Patients whose internal sphincter is known to be compromised by prior TURP or radical prostatectomy should be counseled of near certain stress urinary incontinence after post-RT urethroplasty. Prostate radiotherapy alone likely leads to some internal urinary sphincter dysfunction. The published incidence of de novo incontinence after post-RT urethroplasty is 18.5 % in one series and was associated with urethral strictures of greater than 2 cm in length [50] and 7 % in another with 50 % rate of spontaneous resolution [49]. Using the ventral onlay technique the de novo stress urinary incontinence rate was 25 % [51]. Patients should be counseled regarding the possibility of new stress urinary incontinence after urethroplasty. De novo erectile dysfunction (ED) was reported in 7 % of one series with a 50.9 % rate of preoperative ED [50].

The stress urinary incontinence that results from a post-RT urethroplasty can be managed with the placement of the artificial urinary sphincter (AUS). Typically, the device is placed 3–6 months after the urethroplasty to allow for adequate anastomotic healing and to ensure urethral patency on cystoscopic evaluation at the initial follow up visit. Radiotherapy appears to increase the risk of AUS revision. Bates et al. published a meta-analysis of 1886 patients who underwent AUS after radical prostatectomy versus radical prostatectomy and EBRT. The revision rate was 16 % higher with a risk ratio of 1.56 in the RP+EBRT group with infection/erosion being the major contributors to the increased revision rate [52]. Brant et al. performed a prospective analysis of 386 patients undergoing AUS and found that pelvic radiotherapy significantly increased the risk of device erosion from 3 % in the non-radiated patients to 15 % in those with a history of radiotherapy. A history of prior urethroplasty did not change the erosion rates [53]. The male urethral sling is not recommended in patients after radiotherapy.

Post-operative Surveillance

Due to higher rates of urethral stricture recurrence in the radiated patient, post-operative surveillance after urethroplasty is important. The median time to stricture recurrence in the post-RT urethroplasty series is 10–12 months [49–51]. For this reason surveillance must continue beyond 1 year after reconstruction and patients should be counseled to follow up if obstructive voiding symptoms return.

Several series include their follow up protocols. Palmer et al. recommend follow up at 3–6 months and 1 year postoperatively with evaluation of subjective voiding symptoms, uroflowmetry, post-void residual urine measurement and cystoscopy [51]. Thereafter patients are generally followed annually with assessment of subjective voiding symptoms, uroflowmetry, post-void residual urine measurement and cystoscopy if any of the above measurements are abnormal. Stricture recurrence is defined as the inability to pass a 16Fr cystoscope [51]. Glass et al. recommend a similar follow up protocol with a RUG and VCUG at 3 and 12 months and with uroflowmetry annually afterwards with a peak flow of 15 cc/s prompting further urethral imaging [49] (Fig. 10.3).

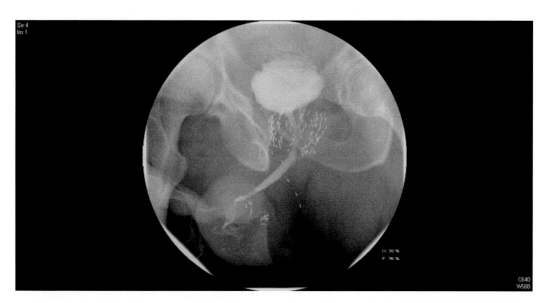

Fig. 10.3 Post-operative RUG/VCUG after anastomotic urethroplasty for bulbomembranous urethral stricture. The anastomosis is widely patent

Conclusion

Post-RT urinary incontinence and urethral stricture disease represent relatively uncommon complications of radiotherapy for prostate cancer however both have the potential to significantly impact the patient's post-treatment health and quality of life. For these reasons a urologic evaluation should be undertaken in patients with persistent or worsening LUTS or urinary incontinence after all modalities of radiotherapy. Medical and surgical interventions can lead to resolution or improvement in both of these post-treatment urinary complications.

References

1. Sriprasad S, Feneley MR, Thompson PM. History of prostate cancer treatment. Surg Oncol. 2009;18:185.
2. Thompson I, Thrasher JB, Aus G, et al. Guideline for the management of clinically localized prostate cancer: 2007 update. J Urol. 2007;177:2106.
3. Thiruchelvam, N., Cruz, F., Kirby, M., Tubaro, A., Chapple, C. R. and Sievert, K.-D. (2015), A review of detrusor overactivity and the overactive bladder after radical prostate cancer treatment. BJU International. doi:10.1111/bju.13078
4. Abrams P, Cardozo L, Fall M, et al. The standardisation of terminology of lower urinary tract function: report from the Standardisation Sub-committee of the International Continence Society. Neurourol Urodyn. 2002;21:167.
5. Abrams P. Describing bladder storage function: overactive bladder syndrome and detrusor overactivity. Urology. 2003;62:28.
6. Antonakopoulos GN, Hicks RM, Berry RJ. The subcellular basis of damage to the human urinary bladder induced by irradiation. J Pathol. 1984;143:103.
7. Marks LB, Carroll PR, Dugan TC, et al. The response of the urinary bladder, urethra, and ureter to radiation and chemotherapy. Int J Radiat Oncol Biol Phys. 1995;31:1257.
8. Lundbeck F, Ulso N, Overgaard J. Cystometric evaluation of early and late irradiation damage to the mouse urinary bladder. Radiother Oncol. 1989;15:383.
9. Choo R, Do V, Herschorn S, et al. Urodynamic changes at 18 months post-therapy in patients treated with external beam radiotherapy for prostate carcinoma. Int J Radiat Oncol Biol Phys. 2002;53:290.
10. Markland AD, Goode PS, Redden DT, et al. Prevalence of urinary incontinence in men: results from the national health and nutrition examination survey. J Urol. 2010;184:1022.
11. Litwin MS. Health related quality of life in older men without prostate cancer. J Urol. 1999;161:1180.
12. Resnick MJ, Barocas DA, Morgans AK, et al. Contemporary prevalence of pretreatment urinary, sexual, hormonal, and bowel dysfunction: Defining the population at risk for harms of prostate cancer treatment. Cancer. 2014;120:1263.
13. Irwin DE, Milsom I, Hunskaar S, et al. Population-based survey of urinary incontinence, overactive bladder, and other lower urinary tract symptoms in five countries: results of the EPIC study. Eur Urol. 2006;50:1306.
14. Resnick MJ, Koyama T, Fan KH, et al. Long-term functional outcomes after treatment for localized prostate cancer. N Engl J Med. 2013;368:436.
15. Sanda MG, Dunn RL, Michalski J, et al. Quality of life and satisfaction with outcome among prostate-cancer survivors. N Engl J Med. 2008;358:1250.
16. Talcott JA, Clark JA, Stark PC, et al. Long-term treatment related complications of brachytherapy for early prostate cancer: a survey of patients previously treated. J Urol. 2001;166:494.
17. Blaivas JG, Weiss JP, Jones M. The pathophysiology of lower urinary tract symptoms after brachytherapy for prostate cancer. BJU Int. 2006;98:1233.
18. Chen AB, D'Amico AV, Neville BA, et al. Patient and treatment factors associated with complications after prostate brachytherapy. J Clin Oncol. 2006;24:5298.
19. Jiang R, Tomaszewski JJ, Ward KC, et al. The burden of overtreatment: comparison of toxicity between single and combined modality radiation therapy among low risk prostate cancer patients. Can J Urol. 2015;22:7648.
20. Gupta S, Peterson AC. Stress urinary incontinence in the prostate cancer survivor. Curr Opin Urol. 2014;24:395.
21. Jeong SJ, Kim HJ, Lee YJ, et al. Prevalence and clinical features of detrusor underactivity among elderly with lower urinary tract symptoms: a comparison between men and women. Korean J Urol. 2012;53:342.
22. Collins CW, Winters JC, American Urological A, et al. AUA/SUFU adult urodynamics guideline: a clinical review. Urol Clin North Am. 2014;41:353.
23. Elshaikh MA, Ulchaker JC, Reddy CA, et al. Prophylactic tamsulosin (Flomax) in patients undergoing prostate 125I brachytherapy for prostate carcinoma: final report of a double-blind placebo-controlled randomized study. Int J Radiat Oncol Biol Phys. 2005;62:164.
24. Zelefsky MJ, Ginor RX, Fuks Z, et al. Efficacy of selective alpha-1 blocker therapy in the treatment of acute urinary symptoms during radiotherapy for localized prostate cancer. Int J Radiat Oncol Biol Phys. 1999;45:567.
25. Bittner N, Merrick GS, Brammer S, et al. Role of trospium chloride in brachytherapy-related detrusor overactivity. Urology. 2008;71:460.
26. Nitti VW, Rosenberg S, Mitcheson DH, et al. Urodynamics and safety of the beta(3)-adrenoceptor agonist mirabegron in males with lower urinary tract symptoms and bladder outlet obstruction. J Urol. 2013;190:1320.
27. Otsuki H, Kosaka T, Nakamura K, et al. beta3-Adrenoceptor agonist mirabegron is effective for overactive bladder that is unresponsive to antimuscarinic

treatment or is related to benign prostatic hyperplasia in men. Int Urol Nephrol. 2013;45:53.

28. Crew JP, Jephcott CR, Reynard JM. Radiation-induced haemorrhagic cystitis. Eur Urol. 2001; 40:111.

29. deVries CR, Freiha FS. Hemorrhagic cystitis: a review. J Urol. 1990;143:1.

30. Tibbs MK. Wound healing following radiation therapy: a review. Radiother Oncol. 1997;42:99.

31. Herschorn S, Elliott S, Coburn M, et al. SIU/ICUD Consultation on Urethral Strictures: Posterior urethral stenosis after treatment of prostate cancer. Urology. 2014;83:S59.

32. Elliott SP, Meng MV, Elkin EP, et al. Incidence of urethral stricture after primary treatment for prostate cancer: data From CaPSURE. J Urol. 2007;178:529.

33. Allen ZA, Merrick GS, Butler WM, et al. Detailed urethral dosimetry in the evaluation of prostate brachytherapy-related urinary morbidity. Int J Radiat Oncol Biol Phys. 2005;62:981.

34. Leapman MS, Stock RG, Stone NN, et al. Findings at cystoscopy performed for cause after prostate brachytherapy. Urology. 2014;83:1350.

35. Merrick GS, Butler WM, Wallner KE, et al. Risk factors for the development of prostate brachytherapy related urethral strictures. J Urol. 2006;175:1376.

36. Zelefsky MJ, Levin EJ, Hunt M, et al. Incidence of late rectal and urinary toxicities after three-dimensional conformal radiotherapy and intensity-modulated radiotherapy for localized prostate cancer. Int J Radiat Oncol Biol Phys. 2008;70:1124.

37. Zelefsky MJ, Yamada Y, Cohen GN, et al. Five-year outcome of intraoperative conformal permanent I-125 interstitial implantation for patients with clinically localized prostate cancer. Int J Radiat Oncol Biol Phys. 2007;67:65.

38. Astrom L, Pedersen D, Mercke C, et al. Long-term outcome of high dose rate brachytherapy in radiotherapy of localised prostate cancer. Radiother Oncol. 2005;74:157.

39. Sullivan L, Williams SG, Tai KH, et al. Urethral stricture following high dose rate brachytherapy for prostate cancer. Radiother Oncol. 2009;91:232.

40. Hindson BR, Millar JL, Matheson B. Urethral strictures following high-dose-rate brachytherapy for prostate cancer: analysis of risk factors. Brachytherapy. 2013;12:50.

41. McDonald AM, Baker CB, Popple RA et al. Increased radiation dose heterogeneity within the prostate predisposes to urethral strictures in patients receiving moderately hypofractionated prostate radiation therapy. Pract Radiat Oncol. doi:10.1016/j.prro.2015.02.010.

42. Lawton CA, Bae K, Pilepich M, et al. Long-term treatment sequelae after external beam irradiation with or without hormonal manipulation for adenocarcinoma of the prostate: analysis of radiation therapy oncology group studies 85-31, 86-10, and 92-02. Int J Radiat Oncol Biol Phys. 2008;70:437.

43. Gardner BG, Zietman AL, Shipley WU, et al. Late normal tissue sequelae in the second decade after high dose radiation therapy with combined photons and conformal protons for locally advanced prostate cancer. J Urol. 2002;167:123.

44. Chism DB, Horwitz EM, Hanlon AL, et al. Late morbidity profiles in prostate cancer patients treated to 79-84 Gy by a simple four-field coplanar beam arrangement. Int J Radiat Oncol Biol Phys. 2003;55:71.

45. Macdonald OK, Lee RJ, Snow G, et al. Prostate-specific antigen control with low-dose adjuvant radiotherapy for high-risk prostate cancer. Urology. 2007;69:295.

46. Cozzarini C, Fiorino C, Di Muzio N, et al. Hypofractionated adjuvant radiotherapy with helical tomotherapy after radical prostatectomy: planning data and toxicity results of a Phase I-II study. Radiother Oncol. 2008;88:26.

47. Chi AC, Han J, Gonzalez CM. Urethral strictures and the cancer survivor. Curr Opin Urol. 2014; 24:415.

48. Erickson BA, McAninch JW, Eisenberg ML, et al. Management for prostate cancer treatment related posterior urethral and bladder neck stenosis with stents. J Urol. 2011;185:198.

49. Glass AS, McAninch JW, Zaid UB, et al. Urethroplasty after radiation therapy for prostate cancer. Urology. 2012;79:1402.

50. Hofer MD, Zhao LC, Morey AF, et al. Outcomes after urethroplasty for radiotherapy induced bulbomembranous urethral stricture disease. J Urol. 2014;191:1307.

51. Palmer DA, Buckley JC, Zinman LN, et al. Urethroplasty for high risk, long segment urethral strictures with ventral buccal mucosa graft and gracilis muscle flap. J Urol. 2015;193:902.

52. Bates, A. S., Martin, R. M. and Terry, T. R. (2015), Complications following artificial urinary sphincter placement after radical prostatectomy and radiotherapy: a meta-analysis. BJU International, 116: 623–633. doi:10.1111/bju.13048

53. Brant WO, Erickson BA, Elliott SP, et al. Risk factors for erosion of artificial urinary sphincters: a multicenter prospective study. Urology. 2014;84:934.

A Case-Based Illustration of Urinary Symptoms Following Radiation Therapy for Prostate Cancer

Allison Polland, Michael S. Leapman, and Nelson N. Stone

Lower Urinary Tract Symptoms following Radiation

Case 1 (This Patient Is 1 Month Post-brachytherapy)

Mr. L is a 72-year-old man with a history of Gleason 3+3=6 prostate cancer (4 of 12 cores, 15 % greatest volume in single core) with a pretreatment prostate volume of 35 cm³and PSA of 4.8 ng/mL. His International Prostate Symptom Score (IPSS) score at baseline was 3. He discussed his options with his urologist and elected for brachytherapy without neoadjuvant hormonal therapy. He completed[125]I brachytherapy 1 month ago, with a minimal dose to 90 % of the prostate volume (D_{90}) of 186 Gy. He presents with complaints of urinary urgency and dysuria.

Lower urinary tract symptoms (LUTS) are categorized as storage, voiding and post-micturition symptoms. Storage symptoms include urgency (a sudden compelling desire to urinate), frequency (a perception of voiding too often), nocturia (the need to wake up at night to void), and urge incontinence (involuntary leakage of urine accompanied by urgency). Voiding symptoms include slow stream (as perceived by the patient or measured on urine flow rate studies), intermittent stream (flow that stops and starts during urination), hesitancy (delay in the onset of voiding), straining (use of abdominal muscles to initiate, maintain or improve stream), and dysuria (pain or burning while passing urine). Post-micturition symptoms include a sensation of incomplete emptying after void and post-void dribbling of urine.

Because patients often experience a combination of these symptoms, urinary symptoms are most often assessed with use of a structured questionnaire. The International Prostate Symptom Score (IPSS) is a reproducible, validated index designed to determine symptom severity. It consists of seven questions related to voiding symptoms. Scores of 0–7, 8–19, and 20–35 signify mild, moderate, and severe symptoms, respectively. In addition, the IPSS includes a quality of life score as a single 7-point scale question asking the patient how he would feel if he were to spend the rest of his life with his current urinary condition (Fig. 11.1). While the IPSS can be used to gauge the symptoms, other primary and secondary tests are often carried out, such as a PSA (Prostate-specific antigen) test,

A. Polland, M.D. • M.S. Leapman, M.D.
Department of Urology, Mount Sinai Hospital, New York, NY, USA

N.N. Stone, M.D. (✉)
Department of Urology, Mount Sinai Hospital, New York, NY, USA

Department of Urology and Radiation Oncology (RGS), Icahn School of Medicine at Mount Sinai, 350 East 72nd Street, New York, NY 10021, USA
e-mail: drnelsonstone@gmail.com

© Springer International Publishing Switzerland 2016
J.S. Sandhu (ed.), *Urinary Dysfunction in Prostate Cancer*, DOI 10.1007/978-3-319-23817-3_11

International Prostate Symptom Score (I-PSS)

Patient Name: _____ **Date of birth:** _____ **Date completed** _____

In the pase month:	Not at All	Less than 1 in 5 Times	Less than Half the Time	About Half the Time	More than Half the Time	Almost Always	Your score
1. Incomplete Emptying How often have you had the sensation of not emptying your bladder?	0	1	2	3	4	5	
2. Frequency How often have you had to urinate less than every two hours?	0	1	2	3	4	5	
3. Intermittency How often have you found you stopped and started again several times when you urinated?	0	1	2	3	4	5	
4. Urgency How often have you found it difficult to postpone Urination?	0	1	2	3	4	5	
5. Weak Stream How often have you had a weak urinary stream?	0	1	2	3	4	5	
6. Straining How often have you had to strain to start urination?	0	1	2	3	4	5	
	None	**1 Time**	**2 Times**	**3 Times**	**4 Times**	**5 Times**	
7. Nocturia How many times did you typically get up at night to urinate?	0	1	2	3	4	5	
Total I–PSS Score							

Score: 1–7: *Mild*   8–19: *Moderate*   20–35: *Severe*

Quality of Life Due to Urinary Symptoms	Delighted	Pleased	Mostly Satisfied	Mixed	Mostly Dissatisfied	Unhappy	Terrible
If you were to spend the rest of your life with your urinary condition just the way it is now, how would you feel about that?	0	1	2	3	4	5	6

Fig. 11.1 International Prostate Symptom Score (IPSS) questionnaire

urinalysis, ultrasound, urinary flow studies, imaging, and cystoscopy. Although cystoscopy is not routinely performed for LUTS after brachytherapy, it can be valuable in evaluating refractory urinary symptoms. In a cohort of 2532 men who had brachytherapy of which 185 men underwent cystoscopy for hematuria or urinary symptoms, while the majority had negative findings, 18 (27 %) had bladder tumors, 18 (27 %) had

hypervascularity, 13 (19.4 %) had radiation cystitis, 7 (10.4 %) had inflammation, 5 (7.5 %) had urethral strictures, and 6 (8.9 %) had calculus disease [1]. Bladder tumors were identified in similar proportions among men with gross hematuria (9.6 %) and refractory urinary symptoms (10.3 %, $p = 0.840$).

Changes in subjective parameters have been shown to correlate with changes in objective parameters after brachytherapy [2]. Maximum flow rate, voided volume, and post-void residual urine volume are decreased at 1 and 6 months after implantation and return to baseline by 1 year. Prostate volume as measured on transrectal ultrasound has been shown to decrease at a year after brachytherapy, although this change is not seen in patients treated with neoadjuvant hormones [2]. Dysuria has been shown to peak at 1 month after brachytherapy. In a series of 581 patients with preimplantation alpha blocker therapy, the frequency and severity of dysuria were found to improve steadily over time with near complete resolution at 45 months [3]. Of the 7 IPSS questions, nocturia and incomplete voiding were found to be the best surrogates for dysuria. Neither clinical nor implant related factors were predictive of dysuria. In a study of 1932 patients treated with brachytherapy alone or with external beam radiotherapy, at 10 years after brachytherapy, minimal change was seen in the American Urological Association Symptoms Score (AUASS), a questionnaire similar to the IPSS. Patients presenting with high initial scores had the greatest improvement from baseline (Fig. 11.2) [4]. Biological effective dose, external beam radiotherapy, hormonal therapy, isotope,

patient age, and prostate size were not found to affect long-term urinary symptoms.

Mr. L had an IPSS score of 18, a maximum flow rate of 8, and a post-void residual (PVR) of 120 mL. He was counseled that his symptoms would likely improve with time and agreed to observation. At 6 months after brachytherapy he had an IPSS score of 8 and at a year after brachytherapy, his IPSS returned to his baseline of 3.

Case 2 (This Patient Is 2 Years Post Brachytherapy/EBRT)

Mr. B is a 68-year-old man who was treated with brachytherapy and external beam radiotherapy for Gleason 4+4=8. He initially had significant dysuria which was managed conservatively and resolved. Two years after completion of brachytherapy his symptoms returned.

Patients treated by brachytherapy have more symptoms soon after the procedure than those treated by external beam irradiation (EBRT) secondary to the trauma of the needle punctures. Early urinary morbidity does not necessarily

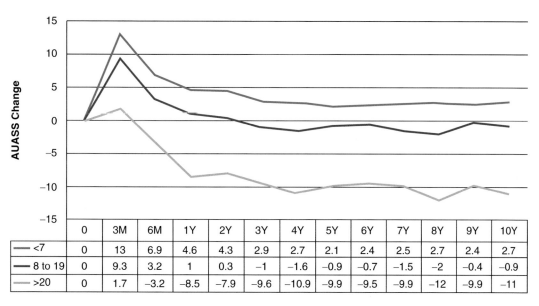

Fig. 11.2 Change in AUASS over time by pre-implant severity category ($p=0.001$ for all points). Used with permission [4]

predict worsened long term urinary function [5]. Urinary morbidity peaks immediately following radiation and then slowly returns to baseline. In a cohort of 1932 men treated with prostate brachytherapy alone or with external beam radiation followed a mean of 6.8 years, AUASS peaked at 0–3 months after brachytherapy implant. This was followed by a steady return to within 1 point of baseline by 3 years (Fig. 11.2) [4]. This study also found that patients presenting with high initial symptom scores had the greatest improvement with an average 11-point reduction in symptoms at 10 years. While many patients have resolution of symptoms after the initial peak, a late worsening or "flare" in symptoms has also been described. This transient late exacerbation of urinary symptoms occurs in over a third of patients by 5 years, most commonly 2 years after treatment. Flare has been defined as a rise in IPSS from the nadir symptom score of at least five points. Neither clinical nor implant related factors have been shown to be predictive of flare [6]. A "PSA bounce" has also not been found to be associated with urinary symptom flare. The patient's symptoms resolved over the following 3–6 months.

Case 3 (This Patient with a Large Prostate is Being Counseled about Brachytherapy)

Mr. P is a 69-year-old man who presented to his urologist with LUTS. The urologist performed a digital rectal exam and found a large prostate approximately 60 g with a nodule suspicious for cancer. Mr. P underwent biopsy which showed Gleason 3 + 4 = 7 with a prostate volume of 60 cc. He was interested in radiation therapy and was curious to know how it might affect his urinary symptoms and quality of life.

Patients receiving radiation therapy may experience urinary symptoms resulting from patient or treatment specific factors. Patient specific factors which can affect voiding symptoms include pretreatment symptom score, androgen deprivation, prostate volume and transition zone index.

Pretreatment IPSS has been shown to be predictive of posttreatment symptoms in a number of studies [6]. Neoadjuvant-hormonal therapy is associated with decreased rate of retention in patients with large prostate glands and IPSS greater than 15 [7]. Prostate volume has also been shown to be predictive of symptoms and hormonal therapy can affect prostate volume [8]. The transition zone index (TZI) is calculated as transition zone volume/prostate gland volume. Transition zone volume may affect LUTS; the TZI has been shown to be associated with urinary symptoms [9].

The most fundamental treatment specific factor is type of radiation. Lower urinary tract symptoms can occur after external beam radiotherapy (EBRT) as well as after brachytherapy. Zelefsky et al. compared men who were treated with EBRT with men who were treated with brachytherapy [10]. In the short term, those who received brachytherapy had slightly higher urinary toxicity (e.g., urethral stricture) compared with those who were treated with EBRT, although urinary symptoms subsequently resolved or improved in most patients. A study of the CaPSURE database, looking at locally advanced prostate cancer found no treatment modality was superior to others based on quality of life outcomes [11].

For patients undergoing brachytherapy there are a number of procedure specific factors that can affect urinary function including isotope type, delivery approach, total prostate and urethral dose, and number of needles and seeds implanted. The two commonly used isotopes for permanent prostate seed brachytherapy are iodine-125 (^{125}I) and palladium-103 (^{103}Pd). ^{125}I has a half-life of 60 days with an average energy of 28 KeV. ^{103}Pd has a half-life of 17 days with an average energy of 21 KeV. There is a theoretical concern that the rapid dose delivery associated with ^{103}Pd could cause increased morbidity in large prostate glands. However in a study of almost 1000 patients, regardless of prostate size, isotope (^{125}I versus ^{103}Pd) did not impact IPSS resolution, catheter dependency, or the need for surgical intervention. Cesium-131, a newer isotope, has a half-life of 9.7 days with an energy of 29 KeV. Cesium-131 delivers 90 % of its therapeutic dose within 1 month. Because it was approved in 2003, there are no long-term studies of the urinary effects of this isotope, but theoretically the faster dose rate could result in a faster resolution of urinary symptoms [12].

There are two main approaches to delivery of prostate brachytherapy: preplanning, in which all calculations are made ahead of the implant date and preloaded needles are used, and intraoperative real-time dose calculation. Intraoperative dose calculation has been shown to result in better gland isodose coverage but is associated with higher IPSS scores after implantation which remain elevated for longer [13]. Total dose and dose-volume factors have also been shown to be correlated with IPSS and within the IPSS, specifically with frequency [14]. Dose to the urethra was found to affect frequency most significantly. The number of seeds inserted has been shown to correlate with increased need for catheterization, although it was not found to be predictive of elevated IPSS [8]. Difficulty of implant, as measured by the number of needles which had to unexpectedly be placed in unassigned coordinates, has also been shown to be associated with need for catheterization, but not with high post-treatment IPSS [8].

Given that the majority of patients with prostate cancer do not die of the disease and there are a number of treatment options for prostate cancer, quality of life after treatment can affect patient decision-making regarding treatment options. In a study looking at the early posttreatment period using the Short Form (36) Health Survey (SF-36), the best general physical functioning was reported by patients who underwent brachytherapy followed by external beam radiation and radical prostatectomy (RP) [15]. With time, quality of life differences between groups lessened. At an average of 7.5 months after treatment the general health related quality of life of patients undergoing brachytherapy with and without pretreatment external beam radiation was similar to age matched controls [16]. At a mean follow-up of 66.3 months after brachytherapy, patients were found to have urinary quality of life scores similar to newly diagnosed prostate cancer patients of comparable demographics [17]. Use of neoadjuvant or adjuvant hormonal

therapy has been shown to have no significant impact on quality of life with no difference in the irritative or obstructive subscales of the AUASS at 24 months after implantation [18].

Case 4 (This Patient Is Being Counseled about Brachytherapy)

Mr. F is a 66-year-old man diagnosed with Gleason 3+3=6. He is interested in brachytherapy but is concerned about developing LUTS. He wants to know if there is anything he can do to prevent the development of these symptoms.

In many reported series, an alpha blocker is initiated before brachytherapy [3]. Alpha-blocker therapy has been shown to affect temporal resolution of urinary morbidity following prostate brachytherapy [19]. A double-blind, placebo-controlled, randomized trial found prophylactic tamsulosin (0.8 mg/day) did not significantly affect urinary retention rates, but had a positive effect on urinary morbidity at week 5 after brachytherapy implant as measured by AUASS [19]. The use of prophylactic alpha blocker therapy was examined in 234 patients including 142 who received therapy prior to implantation and until the return to baseline IPSS levels, as well as 92 who received alpha-blocker therapy only for the occurrence of obstructive urinary symptoms. While patients receiving prophylactic alpha blockers experienced a faster return to baseline IPSS levels, there was no observed difference in the incidence of urinary retention [20].

Case 5 (This Patient with a Prior TURP is 2 Years Post-brachytherapy)

Mr. W is a 71-year-old male with history of clinical T2a, Gleason 3+3=6 prostate cancer, pretreatment PSA 3.9 ng/mL, who received treatment with[125]I monotherapy 2 years ago. Two years prior to implantation he had a transurethral resection of the prostate with 20 g of tissue resected. His PSA is still decreasing at 1.5 ng/mL, but he has experienced progressive weakening of his urinary stream. His

IPSS is 20 and his PVR is 100 mL. A cystoscopy reveals a circumferential proximal (prostatic) urethral stricture.

The occurrence of urethral stricture disease following brachytherapy has been reported in the range of 0–12 % [21–24]. Merrick and colleagues reported a 5.3 % 5-year actuarial urethral stricture rate, which occurred at a median time of 26.6 months [25]. A similar incidence of scarring has been noted following high dose rate brachytherapy, occurring most commonly in the bulbomembranous urethra [26]. Jarosek et al. compared long-term risks of adverse urinary events following prostate cancer treatment, including 14,259 patients with brachytherapy monotherapy using the Surveillance, Epidemiology and End Results (SEER)-Medicare database. The 10-year propensity-weighted cumulative incidence of urethral stricture or bladder neck contracture was 11.9 % (95 % CI 11–12.95) among patients treated with brachytherapy alone, compared with 19.4 % (95 % CI 18.23–20.62) for combination brachytherapy and external beam radiotherapy, as well as 19.3 % (95 % CI 18.74–19.96) for radical prostatectomy [27]. Similarly, a Cochrane systematic database review identified a pooled incidence of stricture in 2/85 (2.4 %) compared with 6/89 (6.7 %) of patients treated with prostatectomy ($p=0.221$) [28].

The appearance of urethral stricture following implantation appears to be influenced by several dosimetric factors including the dose delivered to the membranous urethra. In one study of 1186 patients treated with brachytherapy, 29 developed urethral strictures, this adverse outcome was associated with higher dose to the bulbomembranous urethra (105.6 % versus 85.5 % of planned dose, $p=0.002$) [29]. Patients with radiation induced strictures have been conventionally approached with initial dilation and/or endoscopic urethrotomy. Reconstruction with urethroplasty may be performed for post-radiation strictures with and without tissue transfer. Glass et al. reported on 29 patients with radiation-induced stricture in the bulbous (41 %) and membranous (41 %) urethra using anastomotic, buccal mucosal graft and perineal flap techniques with an overall success rate of 90 % [30]. In a multi-institutional review of 72 cases from 3 academic sites treated primarily with anastomotic urethroplasty, successful reconstruction was achieved in 69.7 %, and incontinence developed in 18.5 %, and was associated with longer stricture length (>2 cm) [31].

There is a distinct difference between post-TURP prostatic urethral strictures and those occurring in the membranous or bulbar urethra. In the former, extra care needs to be taken not to place seeds too close to the TUR defect or bladder neck, while still maintaining adequate dose distribution. In the latter, stricture occurs because of errant seed placement inferior to the prostate apex. This occurs when physicians do not use real-time placement and overcompensated apical coverage.

Mr. W had an incision of the stricture and was placed on CIC daily. Over a 3 month period the frequency of CIC was reduced with complete resolution of symptoms and residual urine. Patients experiencing prostatic urethral strictures with a history of TURP after brachytherapy often redeveloped their strictures following urethrotomy. This is a result of the compromised blood supply from both procedures. A proactive course combining urethrotomy with CIC has been found to be most effective at long term resolution.

Hematuria Following Radiation

Case 1 (This Patient Is 3 Years Post Brachytherapy with Microhematuria)

Mr. O is a 67-year-old male with history of clinical T1c, Gleason 3+4=7 prostate cancer (2 out of 12 cores, 15 % greatest volume in single core), pretreatment PSA 5.3 ng/mL status post[125]I monotherapy 3 years ago. He takes tamsulosin 0.4 mg daily for mildly bothersome LUTS (IPSS 9), and urinalysis sent on workup for urinary symptoms demonstrates 5–10 red blood cells per high power microscopy field (RBC/hpf) without casts, nitrites or leukocyte esterase positivity. He denies gross hematuria. A urine culture is negative. His most recent PSA is 0.4 ng/mL, and digital rectal examination is unremarkable.

Gross hematuria occurring following an interval of normal function post-implantation is a clinically significant event that warrants thorough evaluation. Therefore, most authors agree that patients with any degree of hematuria following implantation should proceed with complete hematuria evaluation. With longitudinal follow, the appreciation for delayed hematuria—both gross and microscopic among men treated with prostate brachytherapy has been described. Hematuria following implantation can be classified by temporal onset: bleeding occurring in the immediate peri-procedural period, and that occurring following a period of normal urinary function (late hematuria). The concern for secondary in-field pelvic malignancy—particularly bladder—following prostate radiation weighs considerably on the occurrence of late hematuria [32].

Reflecting long-standing expert opinion, the American Urological Association practice statement defines microscopic hematuria as three or greater red blood cells seen per high power microscopy field in the absence of a benign cause [33]. Following the immediate post-implantation period, however, it is widely regarded that new onset hematuria should not be merely attributed to an antecedent history of brachytherapy. According to the Radiation Therapy Oncology Group (RTOG), acute gross hematuria with or without clot passage is classified as a grade III toxicity, while hematuria requiring transfusion or bladder obstruction is regarded as grade IV. Similarly, cooperative group common toxicity criteria define microscopic hematuria as a grade I toxicity; gross hematuria without clots as grade II, hematuria with clots as grade III, and hematuria requiring transfusion as grade IV [34].

Barker and colleagues reported on their series from the University of Washington including 215 patients treated with permanent prostate interstitial brachytherapy (^{103}Pd or ^{125}I isotopes) followed for a median of 20 months [35]. Twenty-seven patients were identified (13 %) who experienced gross hematuria occurring 1 week post-implantation. Eleven patients reported one single isolated episode, while the remaining 16 reported multiple episodes. Other publications with longitudinal follow have identified bleeding

occurring at later interval. Anderson et al. reported on 263 consecutive patients who received low dose rate (LDR) brachytherapy monotherapy and minimum of 1 year follow-up between 1998 and 2006 at the MD Anderson Cancer Center, noting hematuria in 13 (10 grade I, 3 grade II) [36]. Larger series with longitudinal follow have similarly identified significant gross hematuria (RTOG ≥ 3) as a rare complication. Keyes et al. reported on 712 consecutive patients receiving permanent prostate brachytherapy between 1998 and 2003 with median follow of 57 months, noting severe hematuria in 0.1 % [37, 38]. However the definition employed in this series addresses only late RTOG grade 3 hematuria, and does not capture the number of patients experiencing lesser degrees of late gross or microscopic hematuria.

We recently published our clinical experience and evaluation of patients receiving cystoscopy for gross or microscopic hematuria. Of 2532 patients, 185 (7.3 %) underwent cystoscopy for hematuria at a median time of 2.7 years following implantation [1]. Most patients presenting with gross or microscopic hematuria had no identifiable pathology on cystoscopy (118, 63 %). The most common findings included bladder tumors in 18 (9.7 %), radiation cystitis in 13 (7 %), and hypervascularity or telangiectasias of the bladder in 18 (9.7 %). Our group has previously reported on a cohort of 2454 men treated at the Mount Sinai Hospital with 5.9 year median follow-up. We identified 218 (8.9 %) who experienced gross hematuria at a median time of 2.1 years, which reflects the latency with which delayed hematuria can be observed [39].

It is not clear whether the incidence of hematuria following brachytherapy implantation is significantly different from observational studies of individuals participating in health screening, which has been cited between 2 and 31 % [33, 40–42]. There is a considerable investigational interest in the factors that predict biological response to radiotherapy, and as a corollary, the factors which predispose to the development of treatment related toxicities. In their 2003 study, Barker et al. reported that hematuria was not associated with patient age ($p=0.4$), pre-implant prostate volume ($p=0.46$), pre-implant American

Urological Association symptom score ($p=0.66$), or maximal or mean urethral dose [35]. However, among our cohort, the development of late gross hematuria was significantly associated with larger prostate size (>40 cm^3), external beam radiation, and freedom from biochemical failure [39].

The occurrence of hematuria following high dose rate (HDR) brachytherapy with 192-iridium has also been compared with LDR implantation using iodine-125 or palladium-103. Grills et al. compared urinary toxicity among patients treated with HDR vs. LDR modalities in 149 patients receiving treatment between 1999 and 2001 [43]. In their study with median follow of 35 months, hematuria occurred with similar frequency in both groups ($p=0.168$), and did not vary by receipt of neoadjuvant androgen deprivation therapy ($p=0.164$). Among 13 of 84 patients experiencing hematuria, all were grade I or II within the HDR group, while all 6 receiving 103-Pd alone experienced only grade I hematuria (Table 11.1).

Table 11.1 Radiation Therapy Oncology Group (RTOG) cooperative group common toxicity grading scale for hematuria

	RTOG [34]	EORTC [44]
Grade I	Microscopic hematuria only	Asymptomatic; clinical or diagnostic observations only; intervention not indicated
Grade II	Gross hematuria without clot passage	Symptomatic; urinary catheter or bladder irrigation indicated; limiting instrumental ADL
Grade III	Gross hematuria with clot passage	Gross hematuria; transfusion, IV medications or hospitalization indicated; elective endoscopic, radiologic or operative intervention indicated; limiting self-care ADL
Grade IV	Gross hematuria with or without clot passage requiring transfusion	Life-threatening consequences; urgent radiologic or operative intervention indicated
Grade V	Death resulting from uncontrolled hematuria	Death

Case 2 (This Patient Developed Severe Unremitting Hematuria following Combination Therapy)

Mr. B is a 63-year-old male with history of Gleason 4+3=7 prostate adenocarcinoma in four out of 12 cores (60 % single greatest core) and a pretreatment PSA of 11.1 ng/mL. He elected treatment with neoadjuvant androgen deprivation therapy (ADT), and palladium-103 implantation with a boost dose of external beam radiation. Following treatment, his PSA nadir is undetectable, and remained stable at 0.08 ng/mL with cessation of androgen deprivation 2 years later. He presented to the emergency room with significant pain and hematuria. A cystoscopy and clot evacuation was performed demonstrating an erythematous, friable mucosa diffusely throughout the bladder mucosa with telangiectasias noted at the bladder neck and trigone area. A biopsy was negative for malignancy but demonstrated obliterative endarteritis, fibrosis, amidst a hypovascular and hypocellular stroma. The bleeding persisted despite continuous irrigation of alum and he required numerous blood transfusions. He returned to the operating room where a cystogram was negative and was infused with 2.5 % formalin solution under general anesthesia. After a 1 month period of response, bleeding continued was refractory to a 10 % formalin installation, and a subsequent 40-treatment course of hyperbaric oxygen therapy. Ultimately he elected a cystectomy with ileal conduit for definitive therapy.

Severe hemorrhagic radiation cystitis following prostate radiotherapy is a rare and challenging complication. In contrast to the acute cellular injury mediated by the delivery of ionizing radiation leading to inflammation and edema, the clinical onset of late radiation cystitis reflects the irreversible damage to vascular and connective tissue [45, 46]. The histological characteristics include obliterative endarteritis resulting in atrophy and fibrosis which is hypovascular, hypocellular and hypoxic. It is thought that hematuria subsequently occurs as the result of necrosis of the hypoxic bladder mucosa, and may also be contributed by the rupture of superimposed dilated blood vessels (telangiectasias). Reflecting the latency of this onset, hemorrhagic cystitis has been observed between 6 months to 10 years following pelvic radiation and the severity classification of hemorrhagic cystitis exists within the RTOG and EORTC genitourinary toxicity criteria for hematuria. At presentation the performance of cystoscopy and biopsy is often required to facilitate evacuation of clot, and exclude the possibility of malignancy.

As illustrated in the preceding case, in addition to supportive care and cystoscopy with electrofulguration, the initial management typically proceeds with instillation of astringent agents to attempt blockage of the site of vascular insult. Aluminum salts (alum) may be administered intravesically following complete evacuation of organized clot at a concentration of 1 %. Aluminum toxicity (encephalopathy and cardiomyopathy) have been reported in patients receiving intravesical infusion, and therefore warrant the monitoring of serum aluminum levels, particularly in patients with renal impairment [47]. Concomitantly, control of bladder discomfort has been approached by many means including intravesical botulinum toxin administration, anticholinergics, sodium pentosan polysulfate, and conjugated estrogens [48, 49]. Formalin, a tissue fixative, has been used after failure of initial agents and following cystographic confirmation indicating the absence of vesicoureteral reflux. If reflux is demonstrated, the ureteral orifices may be first occluded with Fogarty-style catheters. Typical dilutions begin at 1 % and may be sequentially increased to a maximal concentration of 10 % [50, 51]. Irreversible fixation of the urothelium and underlying stromal and muscular architecture can lead to a significant reduction in bladder volume and contractility.

Hyperbaric oxygen is an efficacious therapy with good response rates in cases of recalcitrant radiation cystitis. In-vivo studies of irradiated tissues exposed to hyperbaric conditions demonstrated a significant increase in vascular density which may reflect a macrophage response induced at marked oxygen gradients [52]. In a

series of 62 patients treated between 1988 and 2001, 86 % experienced significant improvement or complete resolution [53]. Prompt initiation of therapy following the onset of hematuria also appears to be a significant factor in response. In a study of 60 patients, 27/28 (96 %) of those treated within 6 months of onset experienced complete or partial resolution of hematuria, compared with 21/32 (66 %) treated at a longer interval ($p=0.003$) [54]. While complete resolution can be achieved in many patients, the durability of these outcomes appears more modest. In a longitudinal follow-up of 11 patients only 3 had complete and sustained response, while the remaining 8 ultimately required urinary diversion as definitive therapy [55].

Following failure of initial conservative approaches, cystectomy with urinary diversion offers definitive therapy by excising the damaged urothelium. The perioperative morbidity and mortality is considerable however, with severe complications (Clavien grade III to V) occurring in 8 of 19 patients, and mortality occurring in 16 % of patients in a series of 21 patients [56]. Supravesical diversions, while sparing the added morbidity of cystectomy, leave the bladder in situ and pose a continued theoretical risk of pyocystis and secondary malignancy and are less favorable.

Case 3 (This Patients Developed a Bladder Tumor following Implant plus EBRT)

Mr. K is a 65-year-old African-American male non-smoker with a significant family history of prostate cancer, biopsy Gleason 4+4 prostate adenocarcinoma (six out of 12 cores, 50 % core positivity), and a pretreatment PSA of 12.7 ng/mL. He elected treatment with trimodal therapy including palladium-103 brachytherapy, neoadjuvant androgen deprivation, and combination external beam radiotherapy. His PSA nadir was 0.01 ng/mL, and is unchanged at 4 years post-implantation. He returns for evaluation following a 1-month history of intermit-

tent gross hematuria; a voided urine cytology is positive. He undergoes cystoscopy with transurethral resection of a papillary bladder tumor. The pathology demonstrates high grade noninvasive urothelial carcinoma and he receives a 6 week course of BCG. He is recurrence-free for 2 years subsequently on surveillance cystoscopy and urinary cytology.

The incremental risk associated with brachytherapy and EBRT on the development of in-field secondary malignancies, particularly bladder cancer, is controversial. Owing to detection biases of patients receiving routine urological care, comparisons to untreated populations may not fully account for the impact of screening. Several recent publications with longitudinal follow-up appear to suggest that pelvic secondary malignancies do occur, but that the risk appears similar to that of surgically treated men. Investigators have compared cohorts of patients treated with radical prostatectomy to matched groups of men treated with intensity-modulated radiotherapy (IMRT) and brachytherapy [57]. Zelefsky and colleagues reported on 2658 men treated with either of these modalities between 1998 and 2001 at the Memorial Sloan Kettering Cancer Center. When compared to radical prostatectomy (RP), brachytherapy was not associated with an increased risk of 10-year any secondary malignancy (89 % versus 87 % $p=0.37$). Among bladder cancers, 4 were detected among 413 brachytherapy patients compared with 16 of 1348 radical prostatectomy patients. In a multivariate analysis adjusting for smoking status, age, and secondary malignancy (SM) stage, brachytherapy as compared with RP was not a significant risk factor for the development of SM ($p=0.83$) [32].

Moreover, the long-term experience has not suggested that bladder cancers that arise following prostate brachytherapy—with or without external beam radiotherapy—are substantively worse or exhibit higher grade features. Of 18 individuals who were subsequently diagnosed with bladder cancer from our cohort of 2532 at a median time of 3.1 years, the majority (72.2 %) of patients had low grade urothelial carcinoma, only two demonstrated muscle-invasive disease managed with cystoprostatectomy. Consequently, there is no current suggestion that patients pre-

senting with newly diagnosed bladder cancers following brachytherapy should receive therapy that differs based on their prior radiation exposure.

Urinary Retention and Transurethral Resection of the Prostate after Brachytherapy

Case 1 (This Patient with a Large Prostate Developed Post-implant Urinary Retention)

Mr. U is a 66-year-old male with clinical T1c, Gleason 4+3=7 prostate cancer in four of 12 cores, pretreatment PSA of 5.5 ng/mL. On his diagnostic transrectal ultrasound-guided (TRUS) biopsy, his prostate volume was 64 cm³ and his pre-implantation IPSS score was 18 with a quality of life score of 3. He elected for iodine-125 monotherapy and was placed on 6 months of neoadjuvant androgen deprivation with an LHRH agonist. At the time of implantation his prostate volume was 40 cm³. The procedure was uneventful and the post-procedure cystogram normal. He voided spontaneously in the recovery room prior to discharge but returned to the emergency room with urinary retention 24 h later. A Foley catheter was placed and he was started on an oral alpha-blocker. After 1 week of catheter drainage, he voided spontaneously and had a post-void residual of 10 mL.

Acute urinary retention (AUR) is a common event following prostate brachytherapy, occurring in as many as 34 % of patients in some series, though the onset and duration may vary [58–61]. The etiology of AUR is generally attributed to obstructive edema of the prostatic urethra, where prostatic volume may increase by as much as 18 % post-implantation [62]. Many clinical risk factors appear to contribute to this outcome including diabetes, larger prostate size, transition zone volume and higher urinary symptom score [63]. Practitioner experience also appears to affect retention rates, possibly reflecting a learning curve in minimizing urethral inflammation [64]. Following catheter placement, the majority of patients experiencing retention will spontaneously void after a short interval of drainage. The addition of alpha blocker therapy, particularly in men with high baseline urinary symptom scores, seems warranted.

The administration of neoadjuvant androgen deprivation in this patient reflects the oncologic benefit born out of randomized evidence in support of a synergistic effect with radiation [65, 66]. In addition to patients with intermediate and high risk disease, we have opted for a risk adapted approach to neoadjuvant ADT. Based on our findings that ADT confers a fourfold risk reduction of retention in patients with prostate volume greater than 50 cm^3 and IPSS >15, it has become our practice to give ADT to these patients [7]. Investigators have also attempted to target the inflammatory response that may underlie post-brachytherapy retention with peri-procedural meloxicam in a randomized trial of 300 patients; however no differences were observed [67].

Patients with persistent urinary retention may be managed with extended catheter drainage, suprapubic tube placement, or clean intermittent catheterization while awaiting resolution of inflammation. The impact on health related quality of life (HRQoL) associated with extended periods of catheter drainage is not trivial. In one study of 127 patients undergoing low dose rate iodine-125 implantation in which AUR occurred in 13 patients, quality of life scores in these patients were lower at study endpoints [68]. Three patients were managed with suprapubic tube drainage and nine ultimately received transurethral resection of the prostate. For men with retention refractory to catheter drainage and medical therapy, transurethral resection of the prostate may be warranted but is associated with a considerable risk of urinary incontinence [69–71].

Case 2 (This Patient Developed Post-implant Retention and Required a TURP)

Mr. G is a 70-year-old male with history of Gleason 3+3 prostate cancer in six out of 12 biopsy cores (50 % in a single highest core), pretreatment PSA 6.1 ng/mL. On TRUS biopsy his prostate volume was 45 cm^3 and a multiparametric prostate MRI demonstrated no evidence of T2 signal abnormality, extra-prostatic extension or restricted diffusion however an intravesical median prostatic lobe was noted. His baseline IPSS score was 8. He elected treatment with brachytherapy monotherapy (iodine-125). His procedure was uneventful, however he was unable to void after catheter removal. No improvement was seen after a trial of alpha-blockers, and a suprapubic tube was placed after 6 weeks of catheter drainage. A urologist performed a limited transurethral resection of the prostate (TURP) (Fig.11.3) and the patient did well after the procedure.

In contrast to transient urinary retention in the immediate post-implantation period, prolonged periods of complete bladder outlet obstruction are less common. Among 3600 patients treated with prostate brachytherapy at the Cleveland Clinic, 60 (1.7 %) required a bladder outlet procedure which included photoselective vaporization of the prostate (PVP) or TURP. Controversy exists in the initial management strategy for men presenting with refractory retention with some authors favoring clean intermittent catheterization as long as possible, while others have advocated for early limited resection in patients unlikely to resume spontaneous voiding [72, 73]. To allow for complete delivery of the prescribed dose, we have recommended a minimum interval of five half-lives prior to surgical intervention which varies depending on the isotope used: roughly 10 months for iodine-125 and 3 months for palladium-103. In our series of 2495 patients from Mount Sinai updated in 2013, there were 79 (3.2 %) men who received TURP at a median time of 14.8 months post-implant [70].

The risk of genitourinary morbidity following post-brachytherapy TURP is not trivial, and may vary by many factors including the volume of tissue resected, number of procedures and surgical technique [74]. The incidence of urinary incontinence has been reported to range from 0 to 70 % [75, 76]. Among more recent series, including our own, rates have been in the approximate range of 25 %–39 %. It is clear, however, that resection should be as minimal as possible with

Fig. 11.3 Cystoscopic view of TURP with limited resection

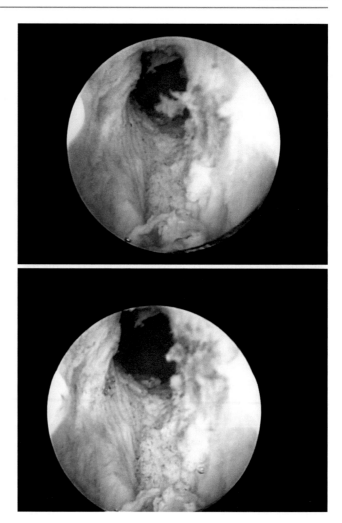

special taken to preserve the blood supply at the lateral and posterior bladder neck. We advocate a very restricted use of cautery and minimal apical resection.

Incontinence Following Radiation

Case 1 (This Patient Had Bothersome Leakage after Seed Implantation)

Mr. M is a 65-year-old male with Gleason 3+4=7 who had undergone iodine-125 brachytherapy 2 years earlier. He presented with urgency and frequency in the morning. He was initially hesitant to discuss it, but after further conversation he also reported leakage of urine.

Urinary incontinence is consistently under-reported by patients, and in some cases denied. In a study of 245 men with early stage prostate cancer awaiting prostatectomy who denied urinary incontinence, a 24-h pad weight test found a mean weight of 4 g (0–35 g) [77]. A history in these patients should include precipitating factors (coughing, sneezing, lifting, straining, changes in body position, alcohol, caffeine, and immobility). It is important to ask about the severity of incontinence which can be measured in number of pads per day and wetness of pads. **Mr. M reported leaking on his way to the restroom in the setting of a strong desire to urinate. Because of this he had begun wearing a pad in his underpants and changed it once each day.**

Urinary incontinence is not a single entity but rather has multiple subtypes with varying causes classified based on symptomatology. Stress urinary incontinence (SUI) is the episodic loss of urine due to increased abdominal pressure as occurs during coughing, sneezing, straining or exercise. SUI may have varying underlying causes including intrinsic sphincter deficiency as may occur with inadvertent damage to the external urinary sphincter during TURP, overflow and detrusor overactivity in which stress triggers an involuntary contraction. Urge urinary incontinence (UUI) is the episodic loss of urine accompanied by a sense of urgency. This may be due to detrusor overactivity; however, low bladder compliance, urinary retention, and irritation due to urinary tract infection may cause it as well. Mixed urinary incontinence is a combination of stress and urge incontinence [78]. Overflow incontinence occurs when a patient is obstructed and cannot effectively empty the bladder; urine may leak out of a full bladder in these patients.

Physical exam in patients with incontinence should start with the genitourinary exam. An uncommon cause of urinary incontinence after radiation therapy to the prostate is continuous incontinence through a urethrocutaneous fistula. In a retrospective study of patients who received radiation therapy from 1977 to 2002, 20 developed urinary fistulae which were presumed to be due to radiation [79]. The majority of fistulae were from the rectum to the urinary tract however three were cutaneous fistulae, all of these patients required urinary diversion for management. Physical should also include a neurological exam to check anal sphincter tone and the bulbocavernosus reflex. Rectal exam may reveal stool impaction. It is also valuable to examine the lower extremities as edema of the lower extremities may create excess urine production leading to incontinence specifically at night when the patient is supine. **Physical exam in Mr. M revealed no suprapubic fullness, rectal exam was normal, and there was no lower extremity edema.**

Initial laboratory studies should include a urinalysis, to check for glucosuria and a urine culture to check for infection. A post-void residual measurement can assess for retention leading to overflow incontinence. A voiding diary, in which the patient records voiding patterns, as well as fluid consumption, may be helpful. Cystoscopy is often unnecessary but could be considered in patients at risk for urethral stricture or bladder cancer, or in those patients in whom surgical therapy is being considered. Urodynamics is also often unnecessary but may be helpful when the diagnosis is unclear. A urodynamic evaluation is often warranted to assess detrusor activity in patients who will undergo reconstructive efforts with artificial urinary sphincter (AUS) or urethral sling. In select cases, a voiding cystourethrogram or spinal imaging may be considered.

The first step in management of incontinence is treatment of possible transient causes. If the incontinence developed in the setting of a urinary tract infection, the infection should be treated. Pharmaceuticals, such as diuretics, should be eliminated if possible. Additionally medical conditions that cause polyuria, such as uncontrolled diabetes, congestive heart failure and lower extremity edema, should be treated. Behavioral modifications such as restricting fluid, avoiding bladder irritants (such as caffeine and alcohol), and elevating legs before bed for patients with lower extremity edema and use of a hand-held urinal for patients with mobility issues may be helpful. Timed voiding may also benefit these patients.

Mr. M had a normal urinalysis and urine culture. After discussing bladder irritants he realized he drank three cups of coffee over the course of each morning. Elimination of these resolved the incontinence.

Case 2 (This Patient Incontinence 5 Years after Brachytherapy)

Mr. T. is a 61-year-old male who had high volume Gleason $3+3=6$ and underwent brachytherapy 5 years earlier. He presented with complaints of urgency, frequency and incontinence. He reported feeling a strong desire to void and was occasionally unable to hold his urine as he rushed to the bathroom. His only other complaint was erectile dysfunction for which he took sildenafil as needed. His physi-

cal exam revealed no abnormalities, urine culture was negative and post-void residual was minimal. He was not interested in medical therapy at this time and was curious to know if there were other options.

Bladder training which involves modification of the voiding interval and urge control can be effective for a motivated patient with sufficient cognitive function to participate in the program. A 2004 Cochrane review found that "bladder training may be helpful for the treatment of urinary incontinence" [80]. **Mr. T tried to void every 2 to 3 h during the day. He also practiced urge control with "quick flicks," contracting the muscles he would use to stop the flow of urine ten times in a row, holding each contraction for 1 s. He returned to the urologist and reported minimal improvement and felt that he was now interested in medical therapy.**

Antimuscarinic agents are the most widely prescribed medication for OAB. They inhibit muscarinic receptors, thereby reducing the response to cholinergic stimulation with resultant suppression of bladder contractions and reduced pressure during bladder filling. M3 receptors are a subtype of muscarinic receptors which mediate smooth muscle relaxation for voiding. There are multiple orally available antimuscarinics. The most commonly used are oxybutynin, tolterodine, fesoterodine, solifenacin, darifenacin, and trospium. Oxybutynin is a nonselective antimuscarinic agent which is also available as a transdermal gel or patch. The main metabolite of oxybutynin, N-desethyloxybutynin (N-DEO), which occurs in high concentration after oral administration, is considered to be the chief cause of side effects such as dry mouth. Extended release formulations and transdermal preparations reduce N-DEO formulation, resulting in decreased systemic adverse effects [81]. Tolterodine is a non-selective antimuscarinic with high bladder selectivity. Fesoterodine is a prodrug that shares its active metabolite with tolterodine but has lower central nervous system (CNS) penetration and less variability in drug availability based on the patient's enzyme activity [82]. Darifenacin and solifenacin are M3

selective agents. Darifenacin has the highest M3 selectivity and does not cause QT interval prolongation which may be a specific concern in certain patients. Oxybutynin, tolterodine, fesoterodine, solifenacin, and darifenacin are all tertiary amines. Trospium is the only FDA approved quaternary amine; it is more hydrophilic than tertiary amines resulting in decreased CNS penetrance [83]. Imipramine is a tricyclic antidepressant which has antimuscarinic activity and directly causes smooth muscle relaxation. It is commonly used for nocturnal enuresis.

Mirabegron is a β agonist that is FDA approved for OAB. It induces bladder relaxation resulting in decreased intravesical pressure during filling and increased bladder capacity, without impairing bladder contraction during voiding. It has been shown to decrease micturition frequency and incontinence episodes.

Phosphodiesterase type 5 (PDE5) inhibitors, such as sildenafil, vardenafil and tadalafil, which are commonly used for erectile dysfunction, have shown symptomatic benefit as compared to placebo in men with lower urinary tract obstruction and resultant lower urinary tract symptoms, such as urge incontinence. They do not affect bladder smooth muscle contractility [84].

Mr. T. was switched from sildenafil as needed to tadalafil 5 mg daily. He was content with his erectile function but still felt that his urgency was not well controlled. He was started on oxybutynin and dosage was titrated up. He denied side effects such as dry mouth and constipation. At 30 mg daily his still complained of urgency and episodes of urge incontinence. He was tried on another antimuscarinic but had no improvement. He considered mirabegron but it was not covered by his insurance. At this point Mr. T was frustrated with his ongoing symptoms despite maximal medical therapy and he was interested to know what other options he might have.

Botulinum toxin acts by inhibiting vesicular release of acetylcholine from the presynaptic membrane in cholinergic nerves resulting in long-term neuronal blockage. Botulinum toxin has been shown to improve urgency, frequency, and cystometric capacity [85]. It is delivered via cystoscopic injection into the detrusor muscle. It is FDA approved for patients with inadequate response or intolerance to anticholinergics, as well as for patients with neurogenic bladder. While there is a growing body of literature regarding use of botulinum toxin in non-neurogenic patients, there currently is no literature addressing its use in the post-radiation population. **Mr. T underwent injection with a total dose of 100 Units, as 0.5 mL (5 Units) injections across 20 sites into the detrusor. His symptoms resolved and he was scheduled for follow-up in 6 months to reassess symptoms at that time.**

Case 3 (This Patient with Irritative Voiding Symptoms Underwent Several TURPs)

Mr. N is a 70-year-old man with Gleason 3+4=7 treated with I-125 brachytherapy implant 3 years earlier. He developed lower urinary tract symptoms including bothersome urgency, frequency, nocturia and incontinence. When questioned further Mr. N specified he had urge incontinence.

While approximately one third of normal older men report some degree of urinary leakage, it is important to determine the cause of the incontinence [86]. Incontinence following brachytherapy is uncommon. A longitudinal study of patients treated with brachytherapy alone found a 1 % incidence of new pad use at 1 year post-treatment [87]. Some patients may develop incontinence immediately after brachytherapy which resolves with time. Anderson et al. found that the number of urinary pads required at 4 months after implantation was no different than baseline, and that incontinence as measured by the Expanded Prostate Cancer Index Composite questionnaire returned to baseline within 8 months of seed implantation [36]. At a median follow-up of over five years, only three patients in the cohort of 263 had incontinence requiring daily pads. Specific risk factors for long-term incontinence in post-radiation patients have not yet been well defined.

Mr. N presented to an outside urologist who performed an aggressive TURP 18 months after implant. He then presented 18 months after this, again with obstructive symptoms and now with mixed incontinence. Brachytherapy in association with TURP has been reported to have varied incidence of incontinence. A literature review found that for patients who had undergone TURP prior to brachytherapy, 0–85 % developed incontinence while for patients who underwent TURP after brachytherapy 0–17 % developed incontinence [88]. In a cohort study of 2050 patients who underwent brachytherapy with or without external beam radiotherapy between June 1990 and February 2004, 38 patients required TURP and seven of those patients (18 %) developed incontinence at a median follow-up of 38 months [69]. Mock and colleagues using the same series of patients with a longer follow-up of 7.2 years found that 20 of 79 patients (25.3 %) developed incontinence after TURP [70]. They found that hormone therapy and number of transurethral resection procedures after implantation of brachytherapy were significant predictors of incontinence on multivariate analysis which included cancer stage, prostate volume by transurethral ultrasound, prostate volume by computerized tomography and total biologically effective dose [70]. In that series, of the 15 patients who required multiple TURP procedures, 8 (53 %) developed incontinence.

Mr. N underwent repeat TURP which showed obstructive scar tissue at apex, which was carefully resected (Fig.11.4). The fluffy yellow tissue seen in the figure, which contains necrotic debris and calcifications, is superficial urethral necrosis that results from over resection and fulguration after high urethral doses of brachytherapy. In the past urologists tended to re-resect this tissue which increased the amount of devascularized tissue. Before recognition of this phenomenon, incontinence rates were as high as 85 % [88]. Understanding this phenomenon has led to lower incontinence rates. **Mr. N tolerated the procedure well and had resolution of his incontinence.**

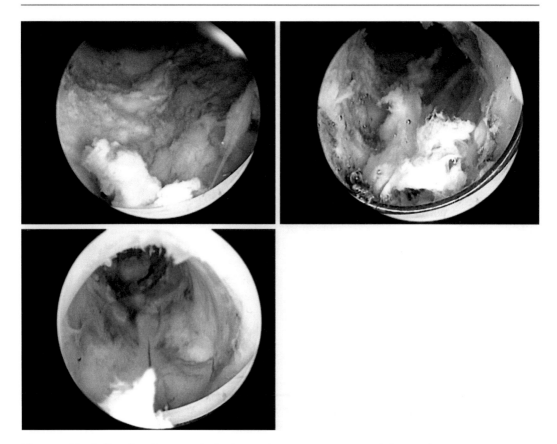

Fig. 11.4 The fluffy yellow tissue seen in the figure, which contains necrotic debris and calcifications, is superficial urethral necrosis that results from over resection and fulguration after high urethral doses of brachytherapy

Case 4 (This Patient Sought Management of Minor Incontinence following TURP)

Mr. G is a 62-year-old man who underwent palladium-103 implant a year earlier and had developed severe obstructive symptoms for which he underwent TURP. Three years later he developed minor stress incontinence when exercising. This bothered him. He had heard about Kegel exercises from his wife and wanted to learn more about them.

Pelvic Floor Muscle Training (PFMT) is a regimen of repeated voluntary pelvic floor muscle contractions also known as Kegel exercises. The mechanism by which these exercises work is unknown although theories include pelvic muscle strengthening and suppression of involuntary contractions. Patients perform isometric contractions of the pelvic floor muscles, holding each

contraction for 6–8 s. A common regimen is a set of 10 contractions three times per day. Patients may have difficulty identifying the muscles to contract, in this case it is helpful to tell them to practice halting urination mid-void which will activate the correct muscles. Biofeedback can be valuable for patients who have difficulty isolating the correct muscles. Sensors are applied to the patient which detect the degree of pelvic floor muscle activity and provide feedback. Other non-surgical options include condom catheters and the penile clamp. Patients who chose to wear a penile clamp should be encouraged to remove the clamp at night as the bladder may become over distended during sleep and excessive compression can cause skin breakdown or tissue necrosis. **Mr. G was not interested in external devices and he did not have success with Kegels. He underwent biofeedback to learn to identify the correct muscles but had no improvement. He** returned to the urologist and underwent cystoscopy. Cystoscopy showed mostly intact but weak sphincter. After discussion of the risks and benefits, Mr. G chose to proceed with bulking agent injection.

Bulking agents are a minimally invasive surgical option. Contigen® (gluteraldehyde cross-linked bovine collagen) is FDA approved for use in men. The ideal patient is one with mild-to-moderate SUI. Patients who have undergone radiation do not respond as well as patients who have not undergone radiation; furthermore continence rates decline over time [89]. **In the case of Mr. G, the tissue below the mucosa was pliable and accepted the collagen injection (Fig.11.5). His incontinence resolved after injection.**

Case 5 (This Patient with T4 Disease Developed Severe Post-implant Incontinence)

Mr. P is a 70-year-old male who initially presented with T4 Gleason 4 + 5 = 9, invading the left levator ani muscle. He underwent a laparoscopic pelvic lymph node dissection which was negative for metastasis. The patient was treated with 3 months of docetaxel and estramustine. He then underwent palladium-103 brachytherapy which included seed implant in the levator ani. Many brachytherapists place implants in the area of the sphincter because of fear of low dose delivery at the apex, this is often not necessary except in the case of locally advanced disease, as in this patient. This was followed by EBRT 2 months later. The patient then received three additional months of chemotherapy after completion of EBRT. He PSA remained undetectable at 10 years after treatment, but he developed stress incontinence. He tried Kegels without improvement.

Mr. P then underwent cystoscopy by an outside urologist which demonstrated a widely patent sphincter due to the high dose delivery to the sphincter which resulted from implanting near this area (Fig.11.6).

Acute urinary symptoms after radiation have been linked to urethral dose, because most prostate cancers occur in the peripheral zone it was at one point hypothesized that urethral sparing therapy could improve health-related quality of life while maintaining prostate cancer control. However a randomized trial demonstrated that urethral sparing radiation therapy failed to improve health-related quality of life and resulted in higher PSA nadir and inferior biochemical control [90].

Noting the wide open sphincter the urologist, who had little experience with post-brachytherapy patients, offered Mr. P injection with a bulking agent. Post-injection images are seen in Fig.11.7. Because the tissue was over-irradiated, it had become stiff and would not accept the collagen, resulting in ballooning of the mucosa alone. Mr. P had no improvement with his symptoms. He was frustrated with the lack of efficacy of the minimally invasive therapy and wanted to know what his surgical options were. A friend of his who had undergone a prostatectomy for his prostate cancer had a sling placed and Mr. P wanted to know if he would be a candidate for this.

Male slings are ideal for men with mild to moderate stress urinary incontinence. Patients who have undergone radiation have higher treatment failure rates [91]. There are two types of male slings, anchored slings, which are sutured to the pubic bone or suprapubic tissue, and non-anchored slings. Men with poor detrusor function who undergo sling placement may have a higher risk of urinary retention than men who undergo artificial urinary sphincter placement. Complications of sling placement include scrotal or perineal pain, urinary retention and sling infection or erosion.

The artificial urinary sphincter (AUS) is an implantable device that keeps urine from leaking by compressing the urethra with a deflatable cuff, thereby preventing the flow of urine. The implant has three main components, a reservoir, a cuff and a pump. When the pump is squeezed fluid is transferred from the cuff to the reservoir, deflating the cuff and allowing for urination. After the period of time required to void, fluid automatically returns to the cuff and restores urethral

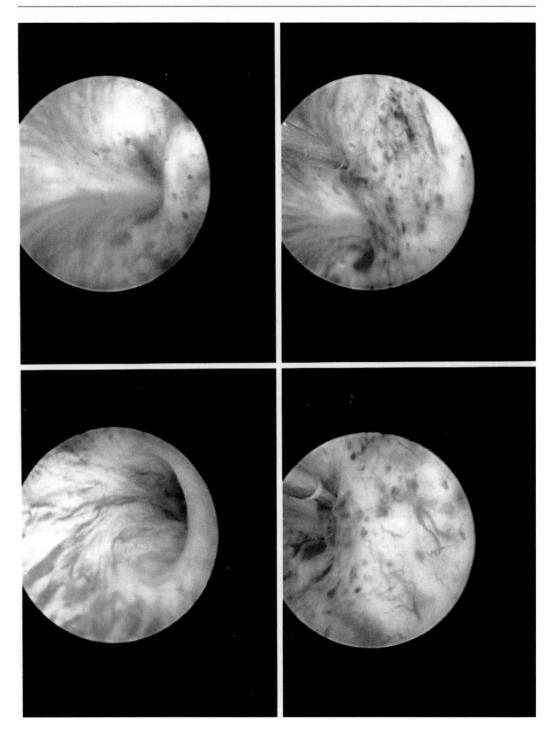

Fig. 11.5 Cystoscopic view of intact but weak sphincter, tissue below the mucosa is pliable and accepts collagen

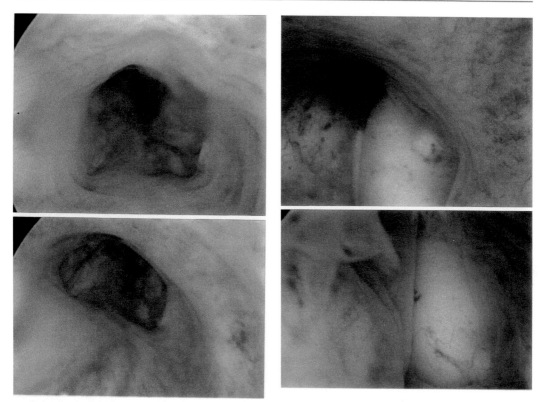

Fig. 11.6 Cystoscopic view of widely patent sphincter

Fig. 11.7 Tissue is over-irradiated and so does not accept collagen injection

compression. Contraindications to AUS placement include impaired cognitive or manual function impeding ability to operate the AUS, unresolved urethral stricture or bladder outlet obstruction, or detrusor overactivity. AUS placement can be performed after bulking agent injection or sling placement. For patients with comorbid erectile dysfunction, a penile prosthesis and AUS may be placed under the same anesthetic. There are few studies discussing placement of an artificial urinary sphincter in post-radiation patients with greatly varied outcomes. AUS or sling placement following prostate radiation increases surgical complexity and evaluation for concomitant urethral stricture disease is also recommended. Rates of cuff erosion and need for revision surgery may be higher in patients with prior radiation, though few studies have specifi-

cally addressed this question in a large brachytherapy cohort [92]. Despite this, it appears that eventual continence and satisfaction rates are similar to non-radiated patients.

Conclusion

Radiation therapy is a valuable tool in the armamentarium of treatment options for prostate cancer. Lower urinary tract symptoms are not uncommon after radiation therapy but often resolve. Hematuria is rarely seen but requires thorough evaluation. Incontinence may be due to stress or urgency and there are multiple treatment options available for each. Understanding the urinary effects of radiation can help us in counseling our patients to better prepare them for their treatment.

References

1. Leapman M, et al. Findings at cystoscopy performed for cause after prostate brachytherapy. Urology. 2014;83(6):1350–5.
2. Tanaka N, et al. Variations in International Prostate Symptom Scores, Uroflowmetric Parameters, and Prostate Volume After 125I Permanent Brachytherapy for Localized Prostate Cancer. Urology. 2009;74(2): 407–11.
3. Merrick G, et al. Dysuria After Permanent Prostate Brachytherapy. Int J Radiat Oncol Biol Phys. 2003;55(4):979–85.
4. Stone N, et al. Factors Influencing Urinary Symptoms 10 Years After Permanent Prostate Seed Implantation. J Urol. 2012;187:117–23.
5. Bittner N, et al. The impact of acute urinary morbidity on late urinary function after permanent prostate brachytherapy. Brachytherapy. 2007;6(4):258–66.
6. Cesaretti J, Stone N, Stock R. Urinary Symptom Flare Following I-125 Prostate Brachytherapy. Int J Radiat Oncol Biol Phys. 2003;56(4):1085–92.
7. Stone N, et al. Does neoadjuvant hormonal therapy improve urinary function when given to men with large prostates undergoing prostate brachytherapy? J Urol. 2010;183:634–9.
8. Kelly K, et al. Prediction of urinary symptoms after 125iodine prostate brachytherapy. Clin Oncol. 2006;18(4):326–32.
9. Merrick G, et al. Relationship between the transition zone index of the prostate gland and urinary morbidity after brachytherapy. Urology. 2001;57:524–9.
10. Zelefsky M, et al. Comparison of the 5-year outcome and morbidity of three-dimensional conformal radiotherapy versus transperineal permanent iodine-125 implantation for early stage prostatic cancer. J Clin Oncol. 1999;17:517–22.
11. White W, et al. Quality of Life in Men With Locally Advanced Adenocarcinoma of the Prostate: An Exploratory Analysis Using Data From the CaPSURE Database. J Urol. 2008;180:2409–14.
12. Jacobs B, et al. Acute lower urinary tract symptoms after prostate brachytherapy with cesium-131. Urology. 2010;76(5):1143–7.
13. Matzkin H, et al. Iodine-125 brachytherapy for localized prostate cancer and urinary morbidity: a prospective comparison of two seed implant methods—preplanning and intraoperative planning. Urology. 2003;62:497–502.
14. Desai J, Stock R, Stone N. Acute urinary morbidity following I-125 interstitial implantation of the prostate gland. Radiat Oncol Invest. 1998;6(3):135–41.
15. Eton D, Lepore S, Helgeson V. Early Quality of Life in Patients with Localized Prostate Carcinoma: An Examination of Treatment-Related, Demographic, and Psychosocial Factors. Cancer. 2001;92(6):1451–9.
16. Brandeis J, et al. Quality of life outcomes after brachytherapy for early stage prostate cancer. J Urol. 2000;163:851–7.
17. Merrick G, et al. Long-term urinary quality of life after permanent prostate brachytherapy. Int J Radiat Oncol Biol Phys. 2003;56(2):454–61.
18. Miller N, et al. Impact of a Novel Neoadjuvant and Adjuvant Hormone-Deprivation Approach on Quality of Life, Voiding Function, and Sexual Function after Prostate Brachytherapy. Cancer. 2003;97(5): 1203–10.
19. Elshaikh M, et al. Prophylactic tamsulosin (flomax) in patients undergoing prostate 125i brachytherapy for prostate carcinoma: final report of a double-blind placebo-controlled randomized study. Int J Radiat Oncol Biol Phys. 2005;62(1):164–9.
20. Merrick GS, et al. Prophylactic versus therapeutic alpha-blockers after permanent prostate brachytherapy. Urology. 2002;60(4):650–5.
21. Albert M, et al. Late genitourinary and gastrointestinal toxicity after magnetic resonance image-guided prostate brachytherapy with or without neoadjuvant external beam radiation therapy. Cancer. 2003;98(5):949–54.
22. Elliott SP, et al. Incidence of urethral stricture after primary treatment for prostate cancer: data From CaPSURE. J Urol. 2007;178(2):529–34.
23. Wehle MJ, et al. Prediction of genitourinary tract morbidity after brachytherapy for prostate adenocarcinoma. Mayo Clin Proc. 2004;79(3):314–7.
24. Zelefsky MJ, et al. Five-year biochemical outcome and toxicity with transperineal CT-planned permanent I-125 prostate implantation for patients with localized prostate cancer. Int J Radiat Oncol Biol Phys. 2000;47(5):1261–6.
25. Merrick GS, et al. The dosimetry of prostate brachytherapy-induced urethral strictures. Int J Radiat Oncol Biol Phys. 2002;52(2):461–8.
26. Sullivan L, et al. Urethral stricture following high dose rate brachytherapy for prostate cancer. Radiother Oncol. 2009;91(2):232–6.
27. Jarosek SL, et al. Propensity-weighted Long-term Risk of Urinary Adverse Events After Prostate Cancer Surgery, Radiation, or Both. Eur Urol. 2015;67(2): 273–80.
28. Peinemann F, et al. Low-dose rate brachytherapy for men with localized prostate cancer. Cochrane Database Syst Rev. 2011;7.
29. Merrick GS, et al. Risk factors for the development of prostate brachytherapy related urethral strictures. J Urol. 2006;175(4):1376–80.
30. Glass AS, et al. Urethroplasty after radiation therapy for prostate cancer. Urology. 2012;79(6):1402–5.
31. Hofer MS, et al. Outcomes after Urethroplasty for Radiotherapy Induced Bulbomembranous Urethral Stricture Disease. J Urol. 2013;191(5):1307–12.
32. Zelefsky MJ, et al. Secondary cancers after intensity-modulated radiotherapy, brachytherapy and radical prostatectomy for the treatment of prostate cancer: incidence and cause-specific survival outcomes according to the initial treatment intervention. BJU Int. 2012;110(11):1696–701.

33. Davis R, et al. Diagnosis, Evaluation and Follow-Up of Asymptomatic Microhematuria (AMH) In Adults: AUA Guideline. J Urol. 2012;188(6 Suppl):2473–81.
34. Cooperative Group Common Toxicity Criteria. Radiation Therapy Oncology Group.
35. Barker J, Wallner K, Merrick G. Gross hematuria after prostate brachytherapy. Urology. 2003;61(2):408–11.
36. Anderson J, et al. Urinary Side Effects and Complications After Permanent Prostate Brachytherapy: The MD Anderson Cancer Center Experience. Urology. 2009;74(3):601–5.
37. Keyes M, et al. Urinary symptom flare in 712 125I prostate brachytherapy patients: long-term follow-up. Int J Radiat Oncol Biol Phys. 2009;75(3):649–55.
38. Keyes M, et al. Predictive factors for acute and late urinary toxicity after permanent prostate brachytherapy: long-term outcome in 712 consecutive patients. Int J Radiat Oncol Biol Phys. 2009;73(4):1023–32.
39. Leapman MS, et al. Haematuria after prostate brachytherapy. BJU Int. 2013;111(8):319–24.
40. Britton JP, et al. A community study of bladder cancer screening by the detection of occult urinary bleeding. J Urol. 1992;148(3):788–90.
41. Messing EM, et al. Home screening for hematuria: results of a multiclinic study. J Urol. 1992;148 (2 Pt 1):289–92.
42. Messing EM, et al. Urinary tract cancers found by homescreening with hematuria dipsticks in healthy men over 50 years of age. Cancer. 1989;64(11):2361–7.
43. Grills I, et al. High dose rate brachytherapy as prostate cancer monotherapy reduces toxicity compared to low dose rate palladium seeds. J Urol. 2004;171:1098–104.
44. Institute, N.C. Cancer Therapy Evaluation Program: Protocol Development. 2009; Available from: http://ctep.cancer.gov/protocolDevelopment/electronic_applications/ctc.htm.
45. Marks LB, et al. The response of the urinary bladder, urethra, and ureter to radiation and chemotherapy. Int J Radiat Oncol Biol Phys. 1995;31(5):1257–80.
46. Smit SG, Heyns CF. Management of radiation cystitis. Nat Rev Urol. 2010;7(4):206–14.
47. Seear MD, Dimmick JE, Rogers PC. Acute aluminum toxicity after continuous intravesical alum irrigation for hemorrhagic cystitis. Urology. 1990;36(4):353–4.
48. Liu YK, et al. Treatment of radiation or cyclophosphamide induced hemorrhagic cystitis using conjugated estrogen. J Urol. 1990;144(1):41–3.
49. Sandhu SS, Goldstraw M, Woodhouse CRJ. The management of haemorrhagic cystitis with sodium pentosan polysulphate. BJU Int. 2004;94(6):845–7.
50. Donahue LA, Frank IN. Intravesical formalin for hemorrhagic cystitis: analysis of therapy. J Urol. 1989;141(4):809–12.
51. Vicente J, Rios G, Caffaratti J. Intravesical formalin for the treatment of massive hemorrhagic cystitis: retrospective review of 25 cases. Eur Urol. 1990;18(3):204–6.
52. Knighton DR, et al. Oxygen tension regulates the expression of angiogenesis factor by macrophages. Science. 1983;221(4617):1283–5.
53. Corman JM, et al. Treatment of radiation induced hemorrhagic cystitis with hyperbaric oxygen. J Urol. 2003;169(6):2200–2.
54. Chong KT, Hampson NB, Corman JM. Early hyperbaric oxygen therapy improves outcome for radiation-induced hemorrhagic cystitis. Urology. 2005;65(4):649–53.
55. Del Pizzo JJ, et al. Treatment of radiation induced hemorrhagic cystitis with hyperbaric oxygen: long-term followup. J Urol. 1998;160(3 Pt 1):731–3.
56. Linder BJ, Tarrell RF, Boorjian SA. Cystectomy for refractory hemorrhagic cystitis: contemporary etiology, presentation and outcomes. J Urol. 2014;192(6):1687–92.
57. Zelefsky MJ, et al. Incidence of secondary cancer development after high-dose intensity-modulated radiotherapy and image-guided brachytherapy for the treatment of localized prostate cancer. Int J Radiat Oncol Biol Phys. 2012;83(3):953–9.
58. Blasko JC, Ragde H, Grimm PD. Transperineal ultrasound-guided implantation of the prostate: morbidity and complications. Scand J Urol Nephrol Suppl. 1991;137:113–8.
59. Lee N, et al. Factors predicting for postimplantation urinary retention after permanent prostate brachytherapy. Int J Radiat Oncol Biol Phys. 2000;48(5):1457–60.
60. Terk MD, Stock RG, Stone NN. Identification of patients at increased risk for prolonged urinary retention following radioactive seed implantation of the prostate. J Urol. 1998;160(4):1379–82.
61. Locke J, et al. Risk factors for acute urinary retention requiring temporary intermittent catheterization after prostate brachytherapy: A prospective study. Int J Radiat Oncol Biol Phys. 2002;52:712–9.
62. Sloboda RS, et al. Time course of prostatic edema post permanent seed implant determined by magnetic resonance imaging. Brachytherapy. 2010;9(4):354–61.
63. Mabjeesh NJ, et al. Preimplant predictive factors of urinary retention after iodine 125 prostate brachytherapy. Urology. 2007;70(3):548–53.
64. Keyes M, et al. Decline in urinary retention incidence in 805 patients after prostate brachytherapy: the effect of learning curve? Int J Radiat Oncol Biol Phys. 2006;64(3):825–34.
65. D'Amico AV, et al. 6-month androgen suppression plus radiation therapy vs radiation therapy alone for patients with clinically localized prostate cancer: a randomized controlled trial. JAMA. 2004;292(7):821–7.
66. Jones CU, et al. Radiotherapy and short-term androgen deprivation for localized prostate cancer. N Engl J Med. 2011;365(2):107–18.
67. Crook J, et al. A phase III randomized trial of the timing of meloxicam with iodine-125 prostate brachytherapy. Int J Radiat Oncol Biol Phys. 2010;77(2):496–501.

68. Roeloffzen EMA, et al. The impact of acute urinary retention after iodine-125 prostate brachytherapy on health-related quality of life. Int J Radiat Oncol Biol Phys. 2010;77(5):1322–8.

69. Kollmeier MA, et al. Urinary morbidity and incontinence following transurethral resection of the prostate after brachytherapy. J Urol. 2005;173(3):808–12.

70. Mock S, et al. Risk of urinary incontinence following post-brachytherapy transurethral resection of the prostate and correlation with clinical and treatment parameters. J Urol. 2013;190(5):1805–10.

71. Merrick G, Butler W, Wallner K. Effect of transurethral resection on urinary quality of life after permanent prostate brachytherapy. Int J Radiat Oncol Biol Phys. 2004;58:81–8.

72. Boone TB. Transurethral resection versus intermittent catheterization in patients with retention after combined brachytherapy/external beam radiotherapy for prostate cancer: intermittent catheterization. J Urol. 2013;189(3):801–2.

73. Stone NN. Transurethral resection versus intermittent catheterization in patients with retention after combined brachytherapy/external beam radiotherapy for prostate cancer: transurethral resection. J Urol. 2013;189(3):800–1.

74. Flam TA, et al. Post-brachytherapy transurethral resection of the prostate in patients with localized prostate cancer. J Urol. 2004;172(1):108–11.

75. Hu K, Wallner K. Urinary incontinence in patients who have a TURP/TUIP following prostate brachytherapy. Int J Radiat Oncol Biol Phys. 1998;40(4):783–6.

76. Koutrouvelis PG, et al. Prostate cancer with large glands treated with 3-dimensional computerized tomography guided pararectal brachytherapy: up to 8 years of followup. J Urol. 2003;169(4):1331–6.

77. Moore K, Allen M, Voaklander D. Pad Tests and Self-Reports of Continence in Men Awaiting Radical Prostatectomy: Establishing Baseline Norms for Males. Neurourol Urodyn. 2004;23:623–6.

78. Abrams P, et al. Fourth international consultation on incontinence recommendations of the international scientific committee: Evaluation and treatment of urinary incontinence, pelvic organ prolapse, and fecal incontinence. Neurourol Urodyn. 2010;29(1):213–40.

79. Chrouser K, et al. Urinary fistulas following external radiation of permanent brachytherapy for the treatment of prostate cancer. J Urol. 2005;173:1953–7.

80. Wallace S, et al. Bladder training for urinary incontinence in adults. Cochrane Database Syst Rev. 2004;1, CD001308.

81. Chapple C. Urinary Incontinence: Oxybutynin topical gel for overactive bladder. Nat Rev Urol. 2009;6:351–2.

82. Mock S, Dmochowski R. Evaluation of fesoterodine fumarate for the treatment of an overactive bladder. Expert Opin Drug Metab Toxicol. 2013;9(12):1659–66.

83. Callegari E, et al. A comprehensive non-clinical evaluation of the CNS penetration potential of antimuscarinic agents for the treatment of overactive bladder. Br J Clin Pharmacol. 2011;72:235–46.

84. Dmochowski R, Roehrborn C, Klise S. Urodynamic effects of once daily tadalafil in men with lower urinary tract symptoms secondary to clinical benign prostatic hyperplasia: a randomized, placebo controlled 12-week clinical trial. J Urol. 2013;189(1 Suppl):S135–40.

85. Popat R, et al. A comparison between the response of patients with idiopathic detrusor overactivity and neurogenic detrusor overactivity to the first intradetrusor injection of botulinum-a toxin. J Urol. 2005;174(3):984–9.

86. Litwin M. Health related quality of life in older men without prostate cancer. J Urol. 1999;161(4):1180–4.

87. Fulmer B, et al. Prospective assessment of voiding and sexual function after treatment for localized prostate carcinoma: comparison of radical prostatectomy to hormonobrachytherapy with and without external beam radiotherapy. Cancer. 2001;91(11):2046–55.

88. Stone N, Stock J. Complications Following Permanent Prostate Brachytherapy. Eur Urol. 2002;50:1–7.

89. Aboseif S, et al. Collagen Injection for Intrinsic Sphincter Deficiency in Men. J Urol. 1996;155(1):10–3.

90. Vainshtein J, et al. Randomized phase II trial of urethral sparing intensity modulated radiation therapy in low-risk prostate cancer: implications for focal therapy. Radiat Oncol. 2012;7(82):1–9.

91. Castle E, et al. The male sling for post-prostatectomy incontinence: mean followup of 18 months. J Urol. 2005;173(5):1657–60.

92. Sathianathen NJ, McGuigan SM, Moon DA. Outcomes of artificial urinary sphincter implantation in the irradiated patient. BJU Int. 2014;113(4):636–41.

Index

A

Abdominal leak point pressure (ALPP), 23, 25
Acute urinary retention (AUR), 7, 44, 160
α-Adrenoceptor agonists, 37
β_2-Adrenoceptor agonists, 37
AdVance sling, 59, 60, 64, 65
Alpha-blocker therapy, 155
American Urological Association score for BPH
    (AUA-7), 21
Androgen deprivation therapy (ADT), 5, 158
Anticholinergics, 6, 95, 142
Antimuscarinic agents, 164
Argus system, 54–56
Artificial urinary sphincter (AUS), 72–74, 76–88,
    93–95, 167
    AMS 800, 71
    in bulbar urethra
        bladder neck placement, 83–84
        closure and follow-up, 81–82
        cuff sizing and placement, 78
        device preparation, 78
        incision and urethral dissection, 77–78
        MS Quick Connect Sutureless Window
            Connectors, 80
        pump placement, 80
        reservoir placement, 79
        tandem cuff, 83
        transcorporal cuff, 82
    device infection, 93
    device malfunction, 96–97
    efficacy and satisfaction rates, 93
    erosion, 93–95
    history and physical exam
        abdominopelvic surgeries, 72
        erectile dysfunction, 74
        hyperglycemia, 73
        manual dexterity, 73
        minimally invasive/open approach, 74
        multicenter prospective study, 73
        SUFU Pad Test Study, 72
    idiopathic leakage, 97
    InhibiZone, 71
    long-term complications
        bladder neck outcomes, 88
        bulbar urethra, 86–87
        mechanical failure, 86
        morbidity, 88
        radiation, 87–88
        urethral atrophy, 86
        urethral erosion, 86
    operative considerations
        rectal injury, 85
        revision surgery, 84
        urethral injury, 85
    perioperative complications and management
        infection, 85
        urinary retention, 85
    persistent Incontinence, 95–96
    post-prostatectomy incontinence
        (PPI), 71
    preoperative testing, 74
    prior incontinence surgery, 75
    revision surgery, 97
    surgical technique, preparation, 76
    urethral strictures/bladder neck
        contractures, 97
ATOMS system, 56–58
AUA symptom score, 142

B

Beta-3 agonists, 142
Bladder neck contracture (BNC), 106
    cold knife urethrotomy, 104
    diversion, 107
    electrocautery/"hot" knife incision, 104
    evaluation, 103
    incidence, 101
    laser urethrotomy, 105
    Mitomycin C, 106
    open repair, 106–107
    presentation, 102
    risk factor, 101–102
    transurethral resection, 105
    urethral dilation, 104
Bone-anchored slings, 62–63
Botulinum toxin, 142, 164, 165
Brachytherapy, 6, 151–153, 155

© Springer International Publishing Switzerland 2016
J.S. Sandhu (ed.), *Urinary Dysfunction in Prostate Cancer*, DOI 10.1007/978-3-319-23817-3

C
Canadian Urological Association (CUA), 23
Cancer of the Prostate Strategic Urologic Research
        Endeavor (CapSURE) database, 4, 5, 102
Clenbuterol, 37
Cryotherapy, 7, 111, 112

D
Darifenacin, 164
Deflux®, 48
Digital rectal examination (DRE), 20, 112, 144
Duloxetin, 37
Durasphere™, 38, 42
Dysuria, 153

E
Electrical stimulation (ES), 35–36
External beam radiotherapy (EBRT), 153–154
External urethral sphincter (EUS), 16
Extracorporeal magnetic innervation (ExMI), 36

F
Fecaluria, 112, 114
Fistulae, 6, 163

G
Gracilis muscle flap, 119–121

H
Health related quality of life (HRQoL), 22, 155, 161, 167
Hematuria, 156–162
High-intensity focused ultrasound (HIFU), 7, 112

I
Imipramine, 37, 164
Internal urethral sphincter (IUS), 16
International Consultation on Incontinence Modular
        Questionnaire (ICIQ), 22
International Consultation on Incontinence
        Questionnaire-Short Form (ICIQ-UISF), 24
International Prostate Symptom Score (IPSS), 151
Intravenous prophylactic antibiotics, 76

L
Lower urinary tract symptoms (LUTS)
    transition zone volume, 154
    voiding symptoms, 151

M
Macroplastique administration device, 46
Macroplastique®, 38, 44, 46–48

Male sling systems
    adjustable sling systems
        advantages and disadvantages, 58
        Argus system, 54–56
        ATOMS system, 56–58
        postoperative pain, 53
        retropubic/transobturator approach, 53
    fixed male slings
        advantages and disadvantages, 64
        fixed compressive slings, 62–64
        retrourethral sling, 59–62
    patient selection, 65
Mirabegro, 164

N
National Health and Nutrition Examination Survey, 4
Non-bone-anchored fixed compressive slings, 63–64

O
Oxybutynin, 164

P
Pelvic floor muscle therapy (PFMT), 166
    Quality of Life (QoL), 35
    randomized control trials (RCTs), 35
    self-directed program, 35
Phosphodiesterase type 5 (PDE5) inhibitors, 164
Post-RT urethral stricture
    endoscopic management, 145
    evaluation, 144
    operative repair, 145–146
    pathophysiology, 143
    post-operative considerations, 146–147
    post-operative surveillane, 147
    presentation and diagnosis, 143
    radiation therapy location, 143
    urethral imaging techniques, 144–145
Posterior tibial nerve stimulation (PTENS), 36
Post-prostatectomy incontinence (PPI), 71
    characterization and LUTS, 19–20
    counseling and treatment options, 17
    cystoscopy, 25
    diagnostic studies, 23
    duloxetine, 17
    early intervention, 16
    imaging, 23
    incidence, 15
    medical history, 19
    pad usage and pad tests, 22
    pathophysiology, 16–17
    patient risk factors, 17–18
    physical exam, 20–21
    quality of life (QoL), 17
    surgical technique, 18–19
    urodynamic studies (UDS), 23–25
    voiding diaries and questionnaires, 21–22

Post-RT urinary incontinence
    evaluation, 141
    medical management, 141–142
    pathophysiology, 139–140
    prevalence, 140–141
Post-void residual (PVR), 23, 126, 131, 141, 142, 145,
        153, 164
Prostate cancer, 4–5, 139
    COLD database, 7
    cryotherapy, 7
    focal therapy, 8
    HIFU, 7
    hormone deprivation, 8
    LUTS, 3
    radical prostatectomy
        anastomotic stricture, 5
        urinary function, 4–5
    SEER database, 8
    TURP, 3
    urinary obstructive and irritative symptoms, 3
Prostate Cancer Outcomes Study, 6, 40
Proximal urinary sphincter, 16

Q
Quality of Life scores, 4, 155, 161

R
Radiation, 6–8, 73, 87–88, 102, 112, 119, 140, 156, 158,
        162–165
Rectourethral fistula, 6
Rectourethral fistula (RUF)
    conservative and endoscopic management, 114
    diagnosis and evaluation, 112–113
    etiology and pathophysiology, 111
    fecaluria, 112
    minimally invasive surgical management, 121
    open surgical management
        gracilis muscle flap, 119–121
        transperineal RUF surgery, 115–116
        York -Mason and Parks Procedure, 115–116
    presentation, 112
Remeex system, 58
Retrograde urethrogram (RUG), 103, 112
Retrourethral sling
    centrum tendineum, 59
    complications, 61
    polypropylene mesh, 59

S
Stress urinary incontinence (SUI), 18, 163
Surveillance, Epidemiology and End Results
        (SEER)-Medicare database, 156

T
Tamsulosin, 142
Terazosin, 142
The International Prostate Symptom Score (IPSS), 21
Tolterodine, 164
Transition zone index (TZI), 154
Transurethral resection of the prostate (TURP), 3, 7,
        165–166
Trospium, 142, 164

U
Urethral atrophy, 61, 75, 82, 86, 127, 128
Urethral cuff erosion, 93, 94
Urinary incontinence
    behavioral therapy
        electrical stimulation, 35–36
        expectant management/watchful
            waiting, 36
        lifestyle adjustments, 36
        PFMT, 34–35
    conservative therapy
        absorbent pads, 31–32
        catheters, 33
        occlusive therapy, 32–33
    Deflux®, 48
    medical management, stress incontinence
        serotonin–noradrenaline reuptake
            inhibitors, 37
        α-adrenoceptor agonists, 37
        β2-adrenoceptor agonists, 37
    urethral bulking agents
        antegrade and retrograde techniques, 38
        antimicrobial prophylaxis, 38
        assessment, 38
        bovine collagen, 38
        injection basics, 39
        injection preparation, 39
        injection technique, 39
        intrinsic sphincter deficiency, 38
        post-procedure, 39
        re-injection, 41–42
Urodynamic studies (UDS), 23–25, 74

Printed in the United States
By Bookmasters